A Field Guide for Setting the Stage

A Field Guide for Setting the Stage

Delivering the Plan by
Using the Learner's Brain Model

Dr. Mario C. Barbiere

ROWMAN & LITTLEFIELD
Lanham • Boulder • New York • London

Published by Rowman & Littlefield
An imprint of The Rowman & Littlefield Publishing Group, Inc.
4501 Forbes Boulevard, Suite 200, Lanham, Maryland 20706
www.rowman.com

Unit A, Whitacre Mews, 26-34 Stannary Street, London SE11 4AB

British Library Cataloguing in Publication Information Available

Library of Congress Cataloging-in-Publication Data Available

Names: Barbiere, Mario C., author.
Title: A field guide for setting the stage : delivering the plan by using the
    learners brain model / Mario C. Barbiere.
Description: Lanham, Maryland : Rowman & Littlefield, [2018] | Includes
    bibliographical references.
Identifiers: LCCN 2018010692 (print) | LCCN 2018026536 (ebook) | ISBN
    9781475841206 (Electronic) | ISBN 9781475841183 (cloth : alk. paper) |
    ISBN 9781475841190 (pbk. : alk. paper)
Subjects: LCSH: Learning, Psychology of. | Learning—Physiological aspects. |
    Brain research.
Classification: LCC LB1060 (ebook) | LCC LB1060 .B3726 2018 (print) | DDC
    370.15—dc23
LC record available at https://lccn.loc.gov/2018010692

For Mom, Dad, and Kermie.

Thanks for your support and love

Contents

Foreword

As an educational leader who has been fortunate to grow up with access to Dr. Barbiere's wealth of knowledge, I have been inspired by so many of his contributions to education throughout my life. As my elementary school principal, from a very young age I learned from him what a true leader looks like when he leads by example and collaborates with the staff relating to his intense wisdom about student learning.

As I began my career as a teacher, it was Dr. Barbiere who inspired me each day to become a better educator. His wide range of expertise helped to guide my pedagogy and instructional practices, especially in the areas of brain research and lesson design.

Dr. Barbiere became a valuable mentor to me on a personal and professional level when I became an administrator. His knowledge of classroom management and how to create an effective classroom climate continues to be an asset to my professional dialogue with educators today. Dr. Barbiere has modeled his practical guide on effective teaching to a colossal number of school districts and classrooms. His knowledge of effective practices has been instrumental for all ethnicities, economical subgroups, and demographics.

Dr. Barbiere has provided an invaluable practical guide to the engagement of learners' brains. He provides teachers with a comprehensive approach to education in the 21st century. He ensures that teachers and students can answer these questions: "Why are we learning this?" and "How will I use this information?"

These two questions tell the student that the material being taught makes sense to them and the value of what they are learning. If the value of the lesson is only for a test, the information may be forgotten after the test. The task instead is for the teacher to help the student see the value of what is being taught, and more importantly, how it can be applied.

Having well-planned lessons will enable teachers to deliver effective lessons and this book's focus is on developing the plan or setting the stage to engage and motivate the learners. The rubrics and strategies in the book have been tested in schools and the feedback was positive. The rubrics are research based so they can be used for coaching purposes or for evaluations.

Setting the Stage: Delivering the Plan by Using the Learner's Brain Model is an essential tool for all teachers and administrators to achieve student growth and teacher effectiveness.

Kevin P. Hajduk, EdS
Principal
John F. Kennedy School
South Plainfield, NJ 07080

Preface

After decades of experience in education and working with many teachers and educators, I discovered that my passion was in school turnaround and student self-regulation. Both cases involved empowerment—in the first case, empowering teachers would make school turnaround permanent and acknowledges that teaching is a dynamic profession in which teachers can continually grow. In the latter, student empowerment encourages students to be self-dependent and not teacher or school dependent.

One way to promote empowerment for teachers and students is to provide rubrics that they can use to assess where they are and what they have to do to improve. For students, rubrics that are standards based maintain standards but lower the barrier as students can assess where they are and what they need to do to get to the next level.

They can self-manage and self-monitor their progress knowing what the expectations are at each level.

Keeping the concept of empowerment in mind, I developed rubrics that can be used by teachers, administrators, parents, or students. I also determined if teachers want to be empowered, they can do peer coaching or peer evaluations. I therefore provided activities that can be done as part of a professional development day to a long-term professional development plan.

The reader will understand how the 21st-century learner needs to be taught in order to self-regulate, become autonomous, and acquire skills needed to become successful in and out of the classroom environment. This workbook will provide you with the toolbox needed to help your students become successful and independent in the future. In addition, this workbook will help you become a master teacher, as it allows you to learn to reflect and evaluate yourself.

The first chapter addresses the planning stage of the Learner's Brain Model and student self-regulation: self-regulation strategies for students when completing home learning, study strategies, organizing their binders, and a student studying checklist for a math test.

The second chapter defines the following areas of lesson design for the Learner's Brain Model: Planning, Instruction, Establishing the Domain, Developing the Essential Question, Planning the Student Learning Target (Objective), and assessing the target via a "Demonstration of Student Learning," which is referred to throughout this book as a DSL. Activities and exercises will be provided for determining if the Demonstration of Student Learning is weak or strong. A rubric will be provided on assessing the objective and DSL.

After the planning stage is completed, the teacher creates the classroom environment—student learning and classroom mood. Instructional practice begins with prepping students by establishing the essential question, developing the Student Learning Target, Demonstration of Student Learning, creating the classroom mood. Instructional practice begins with prepping students by developing a Readiness Set. The Readiness Set gets the student interested at the onset of the lesson. Suggestions are provided for various Readiness Sets. This is covered in chapter 3.

After the lesson is initiated, as discussed in chapter 4, the teacher's task is to develop "sense and meaning" so the information moves from short-term memory to long-term memory. The purpose of developing sense and meaning is to answer the question: "Why are we doing this?" "This doesn't make sense." "When will I use this?" "Will this be on the test?" These kinds of questions are indicative of students not seeing the value of what they are learning, or feeling that what is being taught doesn't make sense to them. Activities are provided to develop sense and meaning because the human brain searches for sense and meaning. Teachers need to offer a variety of approaches and resources to allow for the student to make sense and develop meaning, see patterns for developing relationships, and transfer the new knowledge into real-world application—in essence, the utility of what they are learning.

This field guide can help the facilitator show a relationship between the theory of teaching and learning, and the practical approach of instruction. Teachers, students, and parents will see the relationship between theory and practice. More importantly, they will see how theory can be put into practice. Administrators can use the field guide for a series of workshops during professional development days or for teacher planning periods.

Coaches, resource teachers, supervisors, department chairs, content specialists, behavioral or instructional coaches, interventionists, mentor teachers, peer coaches, district content specialists all can use the information to target specific skills or deficiencies, to model lessons, or as a professional improvement plan resource.

Acknowledgments

There have been many textbooks and field guides written for teachers or administrators to use to improve teaching practice or student achievement. When the underlying assumption is to fix the teacher, that assumption mitigates the power of teachers to problem solve, work collaboratively, or grow professionally. Furthermore, it fails to look at the student and how the student thinks. This field guide focuses on the student because any teacher who has been successful understands the nature of the learner and teaches to the learner. I would like to recognize those individuals who have not only understood this concept but practiced it.

Thanks to Dr. Les Richens, Yasmin Fernandez-Manno, Dr. Peggy Nicolosi, Deborah Bleisnick, Naomi Vilet, and Carol Knower for their County Office support of teachers and administrators as their students reach for the stars. It has been a pleasure working with you.

Special thanks to Sam Garrison and Dr. Pat Mitchell who prompted me to develop rubrics so teachers, administrators, and students can self-assess and monitor their growth. Special thanks to Alice, my wife of forty-four years, for support, encouragement, and love. I love you and miss you.

To all my former Kean graduate students and New Jersey Leader to Leader residents who I have mentored, thank you for helping me grow as a professional.

My family has given me support and encouragement. To Jim, Mairin, Kaleb, Kaia, Chris, Mike, Jackie, and Matt, your support has made this dream a reality.

Special thanks to Alice, my wife of forty-four years, for support, encouragement, and love. I love you and miss you.

Dr. Charles Mitchel, Seton Hall University, Academy for Urban Transformation, has inspired many educators to make a difference in children's lives. He and the faculty of Seton Hall University provide a voice and advocate for many students by developing the next generation of transformative leaders.

Thanks Barbara Bertschy for your friendship and your and Leon Goldstein's support over the difficult times. I'm sure Alice is smiling on us.

Thank you, Carlie Wall and Tom Koerner, as well as Rowman & Littlefield, for making my dream become a reality.

To the teachers, paraprofessionals, staff, and administrators, you are the unsung heroes who go to work every day to help empower students and make teaching a noble profession. The impact you make on your students is powerful and far-reaching. You bring hope for one and all for a better life and a great future. Never extinguish the candle of hope that you bring to light the future. One person can make a difference and that one person is you.

Introduction

This field guide is an invaluable practical guide for the engagement of learners' brains. It provides teachers with a comprehensive approach to education in the 21st century. The field guide ensures that teachers and students can answer these questions: "Why are we learning this?" and "How will I use this information?" The answer to these two questions is that the material being taught makes sense and has the value for application. If the value of the lesson is only for a test, the information may be forgotten after the test. The task instead is for the teacher to help the student see the value of what is being taught (development of meaning) and, more importantly, how it can be applied. One chapter in the book is devoted to making sense and having meaning for the student.

The field guide begins with understanding the Nature of the Learner then moves into instructional planning.

CHAPTER 1: BACKGROUND: THE NATURE OF THE LEARNER: TEACHING TO THE LEARNER'S BRAIN

Knowing how the learner thinks is important. Understanding the nature of the learner allows teachers to construct instructional deliveries or to enable learning to take place to meet the learner's needs. This chapter will provide activities and worksheets for teachers, parents, and students to use for understanding how the brain works. This chapter will also provide handouts, checklists, and strategies for self-regulation, study strategies, homework, or for classroom use.

Directions for using the charts will be provided as well as various checklists for teachers, parents, and students to use.

Focus of the Chapter

Knowing how the learner thinks is important. Understanding the nature of the learner allows teachers to construct instructional deliveries or to enable learning to take place to meet the learner's needs. This chapter will provide activities and worksheets for teachers, parents, and students to use for understanding how the brain works. This chapter will also provide handouts, checklists, and strategies for self-regulation, study strategies, home learning, or for classroom use.

Background

"How does a student learn?" "What is the nature of the learner?" These questions have been and continue to be asked with much frequency. Understanding the nature of the learner is essential, for it allows the teacher to plan effective lessons and to deliver instruction that leads to deep and meaningful learning.

The *teacher* is an essential part of the learning process. Yet, equally important is the *learner* (student). When teaching focuses on the student, the student becomes a self-regulated and an autonomous learner—one who takes control of evaluat-

Introduction Table 1 Personal Strategies for Students to Use to Organize and Interpret Information

Organizing and Transforming Information	Goal Setting and Planning/Standard Setting	Keeping Records and Monitoring	Rehearsing and Memorizing (written or verbal; overt or covert)
• highlighting • outlining • summarizing • rearrangement of materials • flash cards/index cards • draw pictures, diagrams, and charts • webs/mapping	• sequencing, timing, completing • time management and pacing • action plans • set timelines • set short-term goals	• note taking • lists of errors made • record of marks • portfolio, keeping all drafts of assignments • application of suggestions	• mnemonic devices • teaching someone else the material • making sample questions • using mental imagery • using repetition • oral rehearsal

ing and monitoring her own learning and one who acquires a deeper knowledge and higher-order thinking skills. All students, including those from privileged backgrounds, those steeped in poverty, and those in between, must gain their independence from school and become self-dependent.

All students need to learn how to manage and monitor their time, their studies, and their learning, in and out of the classroom, if they are to succeed in school, college, universities, and in their careers. Professionals, teachers, as well as students, need to learn how to facilitate these actions. They need to know how to respond to questions, how to keep the student focused during delivery when the material may be mundane, and how to "kick it up a notch," so to speak, during the lesson.

Research

There is significant research and practical applications of the strategies that were applied for this workbook. By providing the research and strategies, it will enable you, the professional, and those associated with the student, to have the ability to offer strategies and activities for the learner's brain. The reader will learn how the brain works and how the brain switches gears during learning.

The reader will understand how the 21st-century learner needs to be taught in order to self-regulate, become autonomous, and acquire skills needed to become successful in and out of the classroom

environment. This workbook will provide you with the toolbox needed to help your students become successful and independent in the future. In addition, this workbook will help you become a master teacher, as it allows you to learn to reflect and evaluate yourself so you can grow.

This learning field guide is designed to accompany and support the textbook *Setting the Stage: Delivering the Plan by Using the Learner's Brain Model*. The field guide is intended as a tool for teachers, including activities and worksheets for planning lessons during instructional delivery or for student independent work.

Administrators can use the activities for professional development activities, Professional Learning Communities (PLC), grade-level meetings, faculty meetings, or teacher-training sessions.

Students can use the activities to promote self-regulation during instructional class period, independent learning, home learning, or studying.

Parents can use the activities and checklists to help their children develop self-regulation strategies and skills.

This field guide can help the facilitator show a relationship between the theory of teaching and learning, and the practice of instructional delivery. Teachers, students, and parents will see the relationship between theory and practice. More importantly, they will see how theory can be put into practice. Administrators can use the guidebook for a series of workshops during professional development days or for teacher planning periods.

Coaches, resource teachers, supervisors, department chairs, content specialists, behavioral or instructional coaches, interventionists, mentor teachers, peer coaches, district content specialists all can use the information to target specific skills or deficiencies, to model lessons, or as a professional improvement plan resource.

CHAPTER 2: THE KNOWING: PLANNING AND ESTABLISHING FOR THE INSTRUCTIONAL DOMAIN

Focus of the Chapter

The chapter begins unpacking the Learner's Brain Model. Please refer to the text *Setting the Stage: Delivering the Plan by Using the Learner's Brain Model* by Dr. Mario C. Barbiere. The first step of the model is planning/readiness and establishing the learning domain. The role of climate, environment, emotional security, mood, and classroom management are parts of the Learner's Brain Model that will be addressed.

Introduction

This chapter will define the following areas of lesson design for the Learner's Brain Model: Planning, Instruction, Establishing the Domain, Developing the Essential Question, Planning the Student Learning Target (Objective), and assessing the target via an assessment known as a "Demonstration of Student Learning," which is referred to throughout this book as a DSL.

Probing Questions

As a teacher, parent, or administrator, there are questions that should be addressed

1. How does what I want my scholars to know impact my lesson planning?

2. How will I know learning has occurred?
3. What are strategies students can use to self-regulate their learning during this phase?

Lesson Design for the Learner's Brain Model: The Planning Stage

The first phase of instruction is the planning stage. This stage is specifically geared toward diagnosing the data from the previous lesson as well as the information from the formative assessments and checks for understanding that were conducted. The data will determine what should be taught. It involves learning what needs to be done and how instruction should be implemented and delivered.

The first phase of instruction is to **diagnose** the data so appropriate instruction can be planned. Planning guides and checklists are offered for planning a lesson.

Included are: Activities for writing Essential Questions, Student Learning Targets (SLTs), and Demonstrations of Student Learning (DSLs).

What is an Essential Question, why is it used, and how can it be developed? These questions will be developed in this part of the field guide. A template will be offered for constructing Essential Questions, with examples given.

Regarding writing Student Learning Targets (SLT) and Demonstrations of Student Learning (DSL), a template is offered showing weak SLTs and DSLs, and strong SLTs and DSLs. There is also a Reflection Section that can be used for teacher reflection or administrative coaching. Teachers can reflect upon the critical attributes of a strong SLT and DSL, and use the examples of weak SLT and DSL for peer coaching and suggesting ways to improve.

Rubrics for assessing climate and culture, classroom environment, and classroom management are also provided.

Disposition: An effective lesson requires pre-planning so transitions are smooth, student problems are anticipated, and varied strategies are planned to address the anticipated problems.

Lesson Design: The Planning Stage

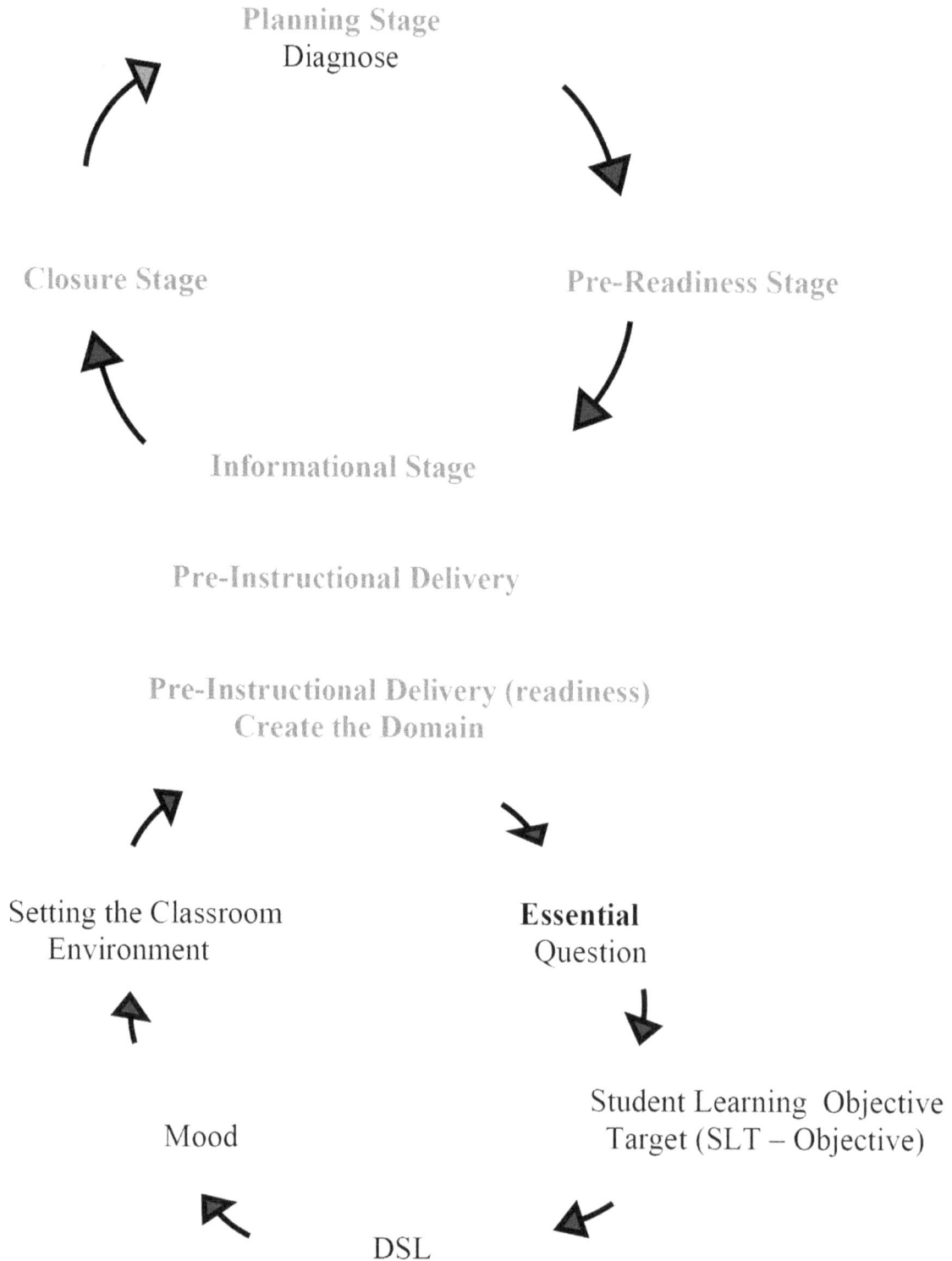

Planning Stage
Diagnose

Closure Stage

Pre-Readiness Stage

Informational Stage

Pre-Instructional Delivery

Pre-Instructional Delivery (readiness)
Create the Domain

Setting the Classroom
Environment

Essential
Question

Mood

Student Learning Objective
Target (SLT – Objective)

DSL

Introduction Figure 1 Lesson design: The planning stage.

CHAPTER 3: USING A READINESS SET

Focus of the Chapter

How to develop a Readiness Set to get the student's interest at the outset of a lesson or at the beginning of a new lesson is covered. After the Readiness Set, the teacher plans the lesson to "make sense" and have meaning for the student. This phase is Stage 1 of the Readiness Cycle.

Introduction

The Readiness Set has three components: the starter (or a catalyst, hook, attention getter); the connection of what will be taught to what students know; and the tie-in of the new information to the student's prior knowledge. Brain research promotes getting the student's attention and holding it, which is one purpose of a Readiness Set. The other purpose of a Readiness Set is to promote sense and meaning.

Probing Questions

1. How will the teacher get her students interested in today's lesson?
2. How will the teacher focus student attention throughout the lesson?
3. What is forward and backward framing and how can it be used in instructional delivery?

Readiness Set

Objective declaration
Forward framing

Sense and Meaning

Introduction Figure 2 Readiness Set.

The Readiness Set has three components: the starter (catalyst, hook, attention getter; sparkler); the connection between what will be taught and what the student knows; and finally the tie-in.

What does brain research say about getting people's attention and holding it?

New brain research increases our understanding of why the Readiness Set is important. Sample lesson plans are provided so teachers can see how Readiness Sets are built into the lesson plan. Additionally, brain research relevant to developing the Readiness Set allows teachers to understand why a Readiness Set is important, and suggestions are provided.

Effective Readiness Sets are provided that are easy to use at any grade level and for any discipline. Specific Readiness Set examples are provided as well as resources.

Use a Song or Video Clip

Description: There are a wide variety of songs and video clips available for use in the classroom. Using songs and clips can be a high-tech way of drawing students into classroom content.

Resources for Creative Starters

www.brainpop.com
www.asset.asu.edu/ (This site is easy to search and offers a wide variety of videos.)
www.thinkport.org/Classroom/onlineclips.tp
http://hubblesource.stsci.edu/sources/video/clips/ (science)
http://www.teachersdomain.org/
http://sciencehack.com/ (science)

There are three components that are necessary for long-term retention: setting the stage with a "mystery," developing a "knowledge gap" (the gap theory between what students know and what they need to know so as to develop their curiosity), and having students predict outcomes. All three are part of the Readiness Set.

This chapter will provide the brain research behind using a Readiness Set and how it connects new information with prior knowledge. There will also be examples of Readiness Sets, and activities for administrators or teachers to use in developing Readiness Sets.

There will also be classroom assessment techniques that can be used to assess the progress of the teacher's lesson. The strategies are useful in monitoring the pace of the lesson as well as in determining the lesson's effectiveness. Based on the information received from the class, the teacher will proceed, pause, and clarify misconceptions, or quit the current direction and adjust the lesson. The teacher's ability to monitor and adjust a lesson is what distinguishes an ineffective lesson from an effective one.

Strategies for students to use in note keeping, which is one part of the self-regulation process, will be shared with examples to use as a template.

CHAPTER 4: DEVELOPING SENSE AND MEANING

Focus of the Chapter

Developing sense and making meaning are required if information is to be stored into long-term memory. Sense and meaning are the "Informa-

tional Stage" of the Learner's Brain Model for Instruction: how to use cues, prompts, reinforcement, and note taking to promote making sense and developing meaning for the student. Activities will be provided to develop sense and meaning.

Introduction

How is making "sense" and promoting "meaning" developed? Why is sense and meaning necessary in the informational stage and for the closing stage? How is sense and meaning developed at each phase of this stage? The various phases in the sense and meaning process will be discussed in the chapter.

Probing Questions

1. What is the role of making sense and having meaning for a lesson?
2. How can a teacher use cues, prompts, and gestures to focus student attention throughout the lesson?
3. What are student "killer questions"?
4. How will a teacher promote reflection to use for student self-regulation?

Sense and Meaning

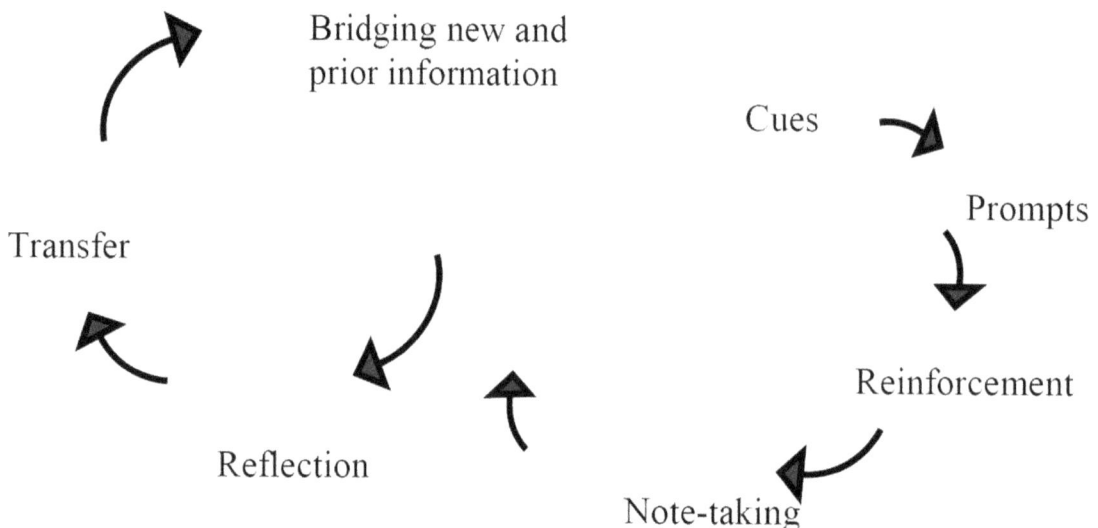

Bridging new and prior information

Cues

Prompts

Transfer

Reinforcement

Reflection

Note-taking

Introduction Figure 3 Sense and meaning.

Sense and Meaning

Sense and meaning are required if information is to be stored into long-term memory. How are "sense" and "meaning" developed? Sense and meaning are also necessary in the informational stage and for the closing stage. How are sense and meaning developed at each stage?

Teachers sometimes hear: "Why are we doing this?" "This doesn't make sense." "When will I use this?" "Will this be on the test?" These kinds of questions are indicative of students not seeing the value of what they are learning or that what is being taught doesn't make sense to them.

This chapter will provide activities for students and teachers to develop the concept of sense and meaning.

There will be strategies included in this chapter for classroom assessment to use for developing sense and meaning, developing reinforcement activities, note taking, and redirection. The critical aspect for development is providing feedback. There will be a "putting it together" section for all of the strategies provided in the chapter.

Research on Sense and Meaning

The sense and meaning question: Why We Are Studying This?

Why are we studying this? Will we be able to use this information? Will this be on the test? These are some of the many questions teachers are asked by students while teachers are presenting lessons. These types of questions send a powerful message to the teacher, which translates into the fact that the student does not see the value or the usefulness of the lesson's subject matter and that what is being taught does not make sense to the student. Additionally, this tells the teacher that the information presented has little or no meaning to the student.

The human brain searches for sense and meaning. Teachers need to offer a variety of approaches and resources to allow for student to make sense and develop meaning, see patterns for developing relationships and transferring the new knowledge into real-world application—in essence, the utility of what they are learning.

How does the teacher facilitate the learning so that the student understands the relationship of the subject matter to his or her own frame of reference? In addition, how will the teacher facilitate the desired outcome, so that this outcome results in students making meaning and a positive connection to the brain of the student?

1

Background: The Nature of the Learner

Teaching to the Learner's Brain

FOCUS OF THE CHAPTER

Knowing how the learner thinks is important. Understanding the nature of the learner allows teachers to construct instructional deliveries or to enable learning to take place to meet the learner's needs. This chapter will provide activities and worksheets for teachers, parents, and students to use for understanding how the brain works. This chapter will also provide handouts, checklists, and strategies for self-regulation, study strategies, homework, or classroom use.

BACKGROUND

"How does a student learn?" "What is the nature of the learner?" These questions have been and continue to be asked with much frequency. Understanding the nature of the learner is essential, for it allows the teacher to plan effective lessons and to deliver instruction that leads to deep and meaningful learning.

The *teacher* is an essential part of the learning process. Yet, equally important is the *learner*. When teaching focuses on the student, the student becomes a self-regulated and autonomous learner, one who takes control of evaluating and monitoring her own learning and acquires a deeper knowledge and higher-order thinking skills. All students, including those from privileged backgrounds, those steeped in poverty, and those in between, must gain their independence from school

and teachers to become self-dependent so they can manage and modulate their learning.

All students need to learn how to manage and monitor their time, their studies, and their learning, in and out of the classroom, if they are to succeed in school, college, university, and in their career. As professionals, teachers, as well as students, need to learn how to facilitate these actions. Students need to know how to respond to challenges. Teachers need to know to keep their students focused during instructional delivery when the material may seem mundane to the student and how to "kick it up a notch," so to speak, during lessons.

RESEARCH

There is significant research and practical applications that were applied for this workbook. By providing the research and strategies, it will enable you, the professional, and those associated with students, the ability to offer strategies and activities for the learner's brain. The reader will learn how the brain works and how the brain switches gears during the learning process.

The reader will understand how the 21st-century learner needs to be taught to self-regulate, become autonomous, and acquire skills needed to become successful in and out of the classroom environment. This workbook will provide you with the toolbox needed to help your students become successful and independent in the future. In addition, this workbook will help you become a master teacher, as it allows you to learn to re-flect and evaluate yourself to improve your plan-ning and delivery.

THE ROAD MAP

The first chapter addresses the planning stage. The subsequent chapters focus on brain research and its implications for lesson planning; how teachers can bring their lesson plans to life; the importance and use of multiple types of assessments before, during, and after instruction; techniques for clos-ing the lesson; and reflecting on the lesson and how to use reflective skills when critiquing your lesson design.

There will be worksheets, activities, checklists, and useful tools for the classroom teacher, admin-istrator, or parent. Please feel free to adapt them to your grade level and your needs.

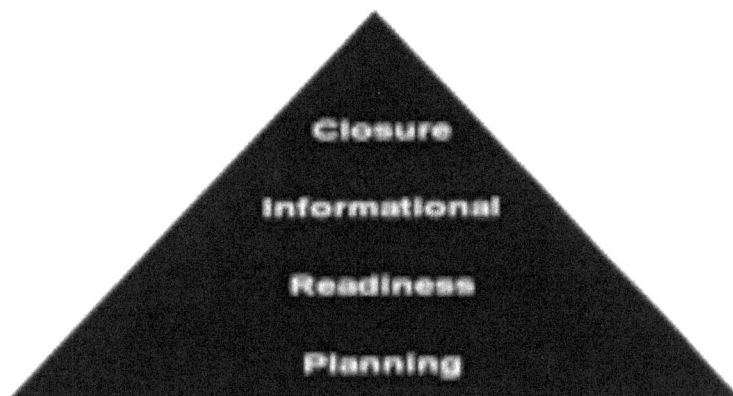

Figure 1.1 The learner's brain model.

QUESTIONS TO PONDER

1. Why is the bottom of the pyramid (planning) wider than the top (closure)?
2. Why is readiness important at the beginning of a lesson?
3. How is information planned to be delivered for meeting the planned objectives?
4. Why is Consolidation for Closure necessary?

Share Your Answers:

Please refer to the diagram that presents a representation of the Learner's Brain Model. Please answer the questions posed then share your answers

Information comes into the brain via the 5 senses.

Once the information comes in from the senses, it goes to short-term or working memory.

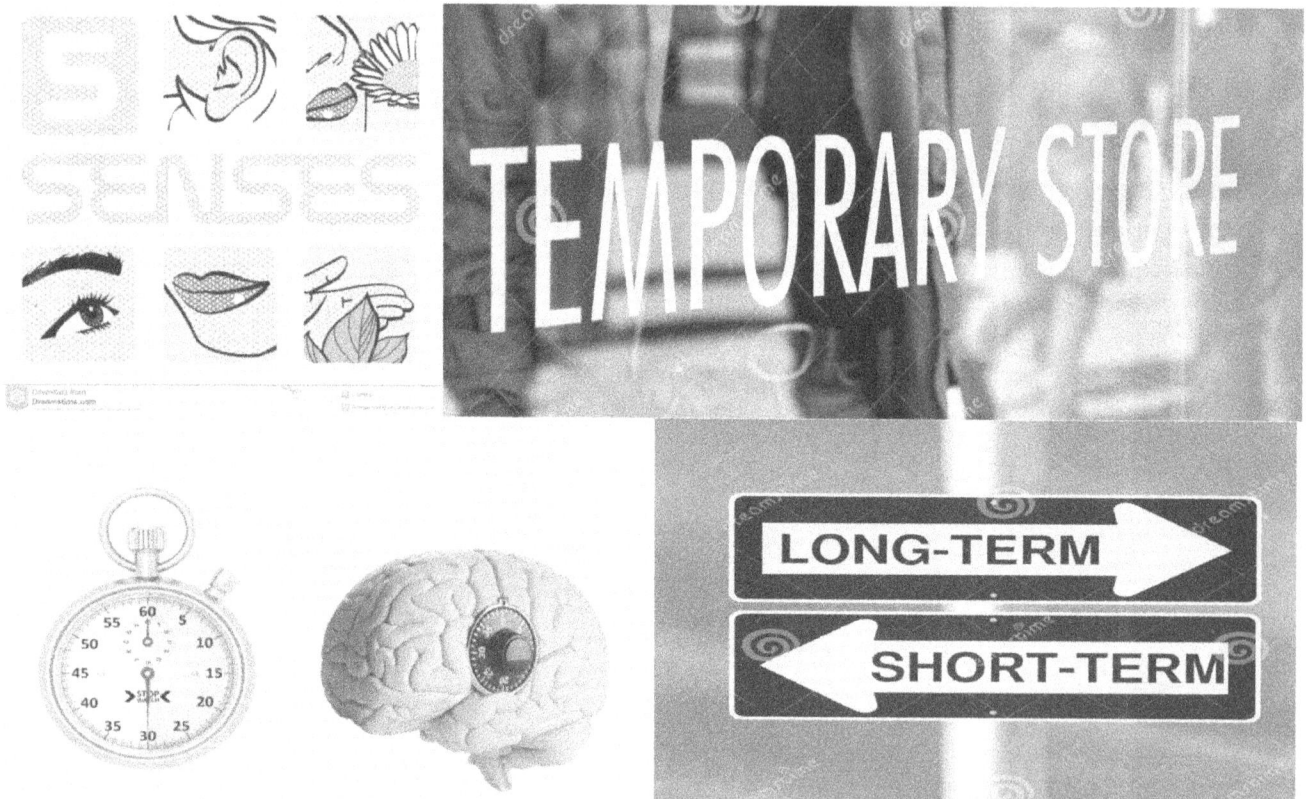

Information stays for 30 seconds.

Sense and meaning is the key for information to get to long-term.

Figure 1.2 A representation of the learner's brain model.

Draw Your Representation of the Learner's Brain:

REFLECTIVE QUESTIONS TO CONSIDER WHEN USING THE LEARNER'S BRAIN MODEL

Lesson Planning and Preparation

Critical attributes: The teacher has extensive knowledge of the important concepts of the discipline and how these relate both to one another and to other disciplines. She understands the horizontal relationships between and among the disciplines. She understands how the relationships among topics and concepts can be linked to ensure student understanding. Teacher uses the nature of the learner, student needs and backgrounds, in planning her content delivery. The teacher determines if the content delivery taught is in isolation or with knowledge of the student's cognitive levels.

Determining the Plan

> **Focus: The teacher must have a depth of subject matter structure and related prerequisites. The critical component of knowing the subject matter and the best-suited pedagogical approach to use when teaching it is based on the nature of the learner. Teachers are teaching students using content not only teaching content.**

- What information will I use to know my students and not your students?
- What do I expect the student to know and do?
- How will I use the Common Core State Standards (CCSS) in planning the lesson?
- How will I extend my content knowledge in the subject/subjects I teach?
- What process will I use as I plan my daily lessons?

- What strategies do I use to check students' prior knowledge and possible misconceptions as I begin the study of a new concept?
- How will I adapt instruction for those students who need extra time and alternative strategies to master a concept?
- What enrichment tasks are available for those who have mastered the concept?
- What artifacts will I collect that will demonstrate student knowledge?
- How will I use student feedback to promote self-regulation?
- Will the lessons be tiered? If so, how will each tier be determined?
- What information from yesterday's lesson will I use?
- What is the essential question I will select? After I select the essential question, how will I tie my Student Learning Targets to the Essential Questions?
- How will I address student learning styles in the lesson?
- How will I scaffold my lesson after my direct instruction?
- How will I plan gradual release?
- How will I promote student self-regulation?
- How will I plan to monitor the lesson?
- How will I plan to close the lesson?

> **Look For: The teacher's plan reflects important concepts and she plans relationships among various disciplines integrating concepts and skills. The teacher has planned her lesson using data, Consolidation for Closure information. She provides clear and accurate explanations with feedback given to promote student learning and student self-regulation.**

Aligning Resources

> **Focus: Teachers align their resources with the learning outcomes and ensure that the resources are challenging to the students as well as appropriate to the students' level.**

- Will a variety of texts and supplemental materials be used, for example, physical objects; math manipulatives or models or science laboratory equipment; print materials, such as maps; primary-source materials; or trade books?
- Will other resources, for example, museums, concert performances, and materials from local businesses, be used?
- Will a variety of resources, for example, internet, library, etc., be used in the lesson?
- Will professional association materials that publish journals or newsletters and sponsor workshops and conferences be used in the planning?
- How will special services be used to support the lesson?

> **Look For: A range of material is available including text and internet, and the teacher encourages students to use all of the resources. Material is appropriate to student reading levels and challenging.**

Student Interest: Creating the Domain

Guiding Question: How will I plan lessons that are based on my students' needs and interests?

> **Focus: The teacher must know her students and plan the content accordingly so one size does not fit all. How will the teacher use her knowledge of her students, for example, cultural heritage, levels of readiness, knowledge acquisition, or identified special needs to plan differentiated lessons?**

- Knowing the developmental characteristics of the age group, how will you plan the lesson?

- How will you learn students' interests and talents so that information can be used in the lesson plan?
- What data will you use to assess students' academic background so lessons can be planned accordingly?
- What evidence will you collect that will indicate student success?
- How will you accommodate students with special needs?
- How will you assess students' progress throughout the lesson and after the lesson?

> **Look For: A variety of sources used by the teacher to acquire knowledge about the students and plan lessons. Multiple projects and options to meet varied student levels are planned. Self-regulation is promoted. Learning needs are incorporated into the lesson plans to address individual student needs. Student accommodations addressed.**

Stage 1: Readiness

The first phase of instruction is to **diagnose,** so appropriate instruction can be planned. What needs to be done and how will instruction be delivered? Once those questions are answered, the first step to planning for the Readiness Stage is establishing the domain.

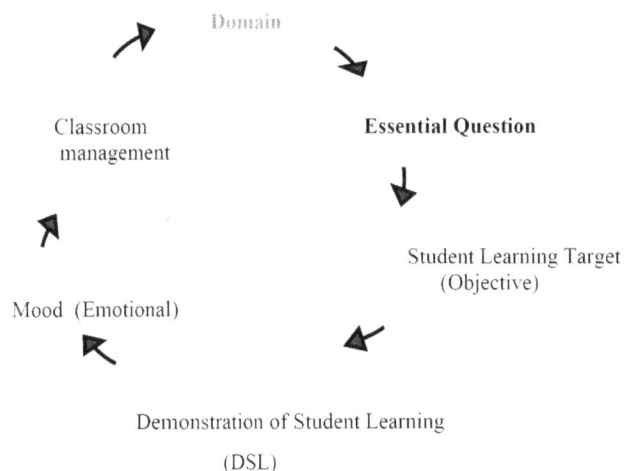

Figure 1.3 Establishing the domain.

Activity

What role does climate, environment, emotional security, mood, and classroom management have in addressing the objective and what are brain-based strategies for establishing each?

How are the components tied together?

Group Findings

The Readiness Set has three components: the starter (catalyst, hook, attention getter sparkler); the connection between what will be taught to what they know; and finally the tie-in.

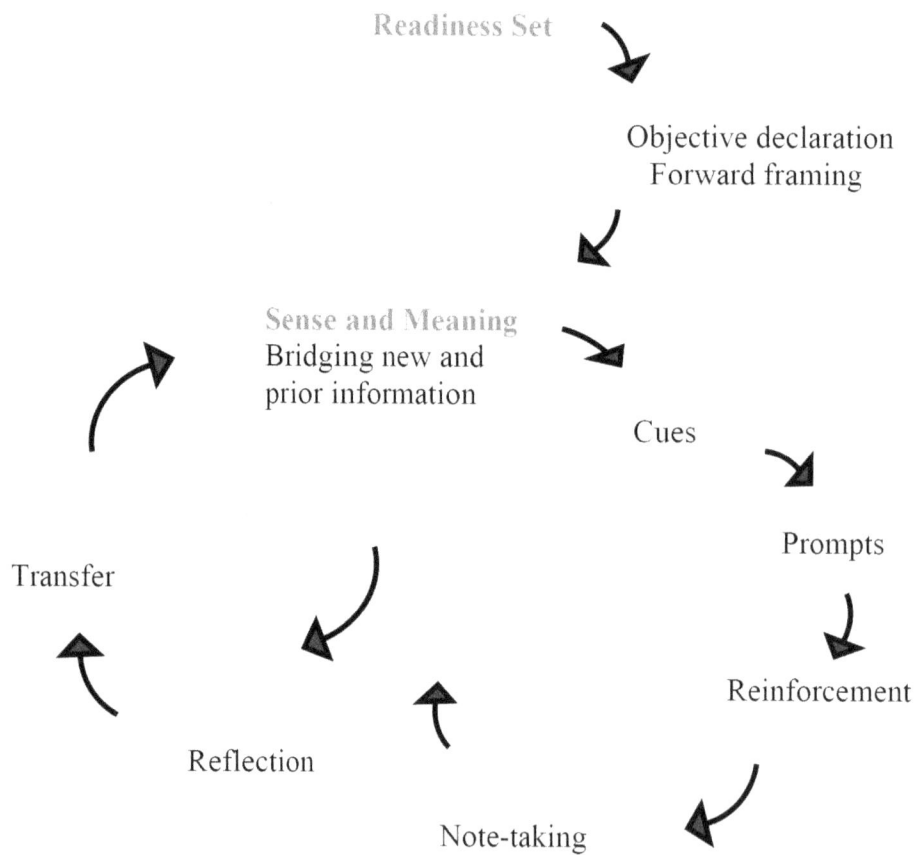

Readiness Set

Objective declaration
Forward framing

Sense and Meaning
Bridging new and
prior information

Cues

Prompts

Transfer

Reinforcement

Reflection

Note-taking

Figure 1.4 The Readiness Set.

As a group, discuss the schema above. Makes notes and share your findings.

Cues

Prompts

Reinforcement

Note taking

Sense and meaning

Findings

Self-Regulation

The most important skill that educators can develop in students is the ability of students to control aspects of their learning. Student self-regulation is one way to control aspects of their learning and for students to take ownership. Without this ability, the students are teacher dependent and not self-dependent.

A self-dependent student has the ability to monitor and control her own behavior, emotions, or thoughts, and is able to alter these based on the demands/conditions of the situation. They can self-monitor and modulate their own learning. This includes the ability to inhibit reactive initial responses, to resist interference from irrelevant stimulation, and to persist with relevant tasks to achieve a goal.

Below is a checklist for students to use when completing home learning.

✓ **Self-Regulated Learning Strategies for Students to Use When Completing Home-Learning Work**

1. Write your home-learning work down in an assignment book so you can monitor your progress and check off work that is completed. All the assignments listed in your book can be thought of as "long-term" goals. Each daily assignment listed for each discipline can be thought of as a "short-term" goal. Check off each assignment when it is completed.

2. Before you begin your assignment, know what is expected to complete the assignment so your work is focused.

3. Make sure you understand the home-learning work before you get home, if not, ask the teacher to explain. Once you get home, if someone is helping you, explain the assignment to that person.

4. Put your completed home-learning work in your homework folder.

5. Develop a schedule for when you will do your home-learning work. Some students like to do their home-learning work as soon as they get home, while others have a specific time.

6. Do your home-learning work in a place where you can concentrate.

7. Have a plan for completing long assignments and projects. Establish benchmarks for completion of the project so you are not trying to do it all the day before the assignment is due. Planning is the most important aspect for long-term assignments.

8. Make sure you have all the supplies and resources you need before you begin the assignment so you do not interrupt your stream of conscientious as you are doing the assignment.

9. If there are directions for completing the assignment, read the directions carefully before you begin.

10. If you do not understand the assignment, ask your parent for help or call a classmate. Make a note of the problem so you can discuss it with the teacher the next day.

11. Focus your attention on doing your best work. Think positive.

12. Take a short break if you have been working for more than 20 minutes. You can try going for a short walk.

13. If you have to go visit someone, bring your home learning with you and complete it in the study area of your new surroundings.

14. If studying, use study strategies that your teacher taught you. (See study strategies, below.)

15. After you complete the assignment, look over the completed work and/or have your parent review it. You can "teach" your parent what you had done as a way to reinforce the learning.

16. Put your completed home learning in your home learning folder and into your backpack.

17. Read for at least 20 minutes a night. (Reading before bedtime is a good way to relax before going to bed.)

✓ **Study Strategies**

1. Chunking—It is easier to remember information when you break it into small chunks. That is why a telephone number is a series of three numbers, three numbers, and four numbers as opposed to a string of ten numbers.
2. Understanding Why—Try to understand information by relating it to your life experience. Ask "why" questions after you read the assignment. Why did that happen? Why does it work?
3. Graphic Organizers—Use visual tools to help you organize information. There are various types of graphic organizers to use.
4. Visualization—Think about what you are learning and then visualize it.
5. Association—Connect what you are trying to learn with a person, place, thing, feeling, or situation. Associations are what some folks use to remember people, as they associate something with the person's name to help them remember the name.
6. Rhyming—Make up a rhyme to help you remember what you are studying. Attach the rhyme to a jingle. The jingle "Nationwide is on your side" is one way to help you remember.
7. Talk—Talk or retell what you are trying to remember.
8. Storytelling—Write a story about the key points you are trying to remember.
9. Writing Sentences—To remember the lines of a staff which are E,G,B,D,F, one can write "Every Good Boy Does Fine."
10. Acronyms—Make up a word from the first letters of words.
11. Rehearsing—Use the VAKT method (Visual, Auditory, Kinesthetic, and Tactile) to practice rehearsal.
12. Mnemonic—A device such as a pattern of letters, ideas, or associations that assists in remembering something.

Strategies for Students

Self-regulation strategies that are most often used by successful students fall into three categories: personal, behavioral, and environmental.

Personal strategies involve how the students organize and interpret information.

Organizing and Transforming Information	*Goal Setting and Planning/Standard Setting*	*Keeping Records and Monitoring*	*Rehearsing and memorizing (written or verbal; overt or covert)*
-highlighting key or common words or phrases -outlining a text to establish key points -summarizing material -rearrangement of information into logical groups -use flash cards/index cards to list key words or phrases -draw pictures, diagrams and/or make charts to have different representations of material -use webs or maps -use graphic organizers -understand purpose or why something is being said or happening -categorize information	-sequencing large projects into manageable sections -establishing a timeline, -establishing a time frame to complete an assignment to help you focus on the use your time -set reasonable goals -develop a pacing chart for long term projects -set benchmarks -set short term goals which are reasonable by working backwards from the due date.	-use journaling to keep a record of how much time you spent on a project so you can budget accordingly for future projects. Make notes in your journal which you will be able to refer back to in the future -make a list of errors so you know where you had problems -record what worked -keep a portfolio so you can document progress, -keep drafts of assignments so you can show your teacher your progress	-use mnemonic devices -teach someone else the material -use oral rehearsal as a way to review material -develop sample questions as a way to help review the material. -use why questions to help promote understanding, make and develop meaning. -develop questions you would use for a test as that helps you frame what is important -use mental imagery -practice using repetition but make sure you use "perfect" practice. -ask "why" questions throughout your study

Behavioral strategies involving student actions.

Self-evaluating (checking quality or progress)	Outcomes/consequences
-task analysis (What does the teacher want me to do?) -did I accomplish what the teacher wanted me to do? -what do I want out of the task? -what will be the gain? -review instructions to make sure the final project meets the criteria of the assignment -provide feedback to yourself using rubrics to assess your work -use exemplars to judge your work. -use standards to judge your work	-the danger of extrinsic rewards is that the behavior may stop when the reward ends. -intrinsic rewards are longer lasting and consistent with student self-regulation and self efficacy -self-reinforcement promotes student empowerment and not student enabling -feedback is needed for improvement. Honest feedback based on standards or rubrics tells one what needs to be done and how it can be done. -feedback based on standards avoids the appearance of bias.

Environmental strategies involve seeking assistance and structuring of the physical study environment.

Seeking information	Environmental structuring	Seeking assistance
-library resources -internet resources -peers -textbooks -journals -books -webcasts -adults	-selecting or arranging the physical setting to promote regulation -isolating/eliminating and minimizing distractions -establishing resource centers throughout the classroom -establishing a "study area" to work quietly -post rubrics and examples	-from your parents -from your peers -from teachers or other adults -exemplary models -from care takers

✓ **High School Student Home-Learning Checklist**

Readiness

- Gather your home learning assignments and all the materials necessary to do the assignment so you don't have to look for material after you get started. Having a break or interruption will require additional time to get back into the "groove" of the work.
- Set specific goals for yourself for each assignment. Having a goal will give you a target to work toward and make the work seem manageable.
- Make sure you have a quiet workspace free from any distractions. Television, telephone, siblings, etc., may be a distraction and make the task much longer and not as effective.
- Make sure you have a clean desk or table—organize your space.
- Begin assignment and take a break every 15 to 20 minutes. Get up and use the bathroom, get a drink/snack, or go for a short walk.
- Review your work as you are proceeding with the assignment and then continue after the review.
- Check in with an adult or older sibling for help if necessary.
- Keep track of your time—use a timer.
- Evaluate your work when you have finished. Use rubrics or exemplars for specific frame of reference.
- Have a parent/guardian or older sibling review your assignments. You can practice oral rehearsal by explaining the assignment to your parent/guardian or older sibling. If you do not have an older sibling, teach your work to a younger sibling.
- Make necessary changes or modifications to your work as needed.

- Reflect on whether or not you met your goals. Reflect on the process you used, how successful it was, what you would change next time, and what worked. List delta and pluses for the experience.
- Grade your work, then compare the teacher grade with your grade to see where you were high or low.
- Submit your work to your teacher to get feedback.

✓ **Self-Regulation for Students Working on a Project**

Before I Begin I Think to Myself:

- What is the project or task asking?
- What do I hope to achieve?
- What strategies do I need to execute to achieve it?
- How much time will this take? Did I set enough time to complete the task?
- What materials do I need before I begin and while I am working on the task?

While I Am Working I Think to Myself:

- Do I understand what I am doing? The task is not to complete a project but to understand the concepts and skills that I am being asked to learn.
- Do I have a series of checkpoints that I'm following? If not, should I establish checkpoints for the project?
- As I am progressing, am I monitoring my work to determine if I need to change any part of my plan?
- How will I know if I am progressing at a satisfactory pace? If the pace is too slow, what problems did I encounter that I have to plan for the next time I do the activity?

✓ **Student Self-Regulation Checklist**

How to Keep an Organized Binder

Organizing the binder

- What is the purpose of keeping a binder?
- How will I organize my binder to address the purpose I am seeking?
- Do I have all the tools necessary to organize my binder, such as paper and tab dividers? If not, will I have the resources to secure what I need?
- Will I have a section for rubrics and exemplars?
- Are the sections of my binder labeled as required? Are they in a logical order?
- Does each section of my binder contain only the appropriate material?
- How often will I go through it to make sure that all the material is in the appropriate section?
- Did I share my binder's organization with the teacher to get feedback?
- Did I share my binder with my friends to get their input?
- Will I have a section in the binder for reflection?
- How often will I reorganize my binder?
- What strategies am I using to keep my binder organized so I do not have to keep reorganizing it?

Reflective Question to Ask as I Work on My Assignments

- Am I reaching my goal? How do I know?
- What is working for me so I can continue the same strategies for other assignments?
- What difficulties am I facing? What will I do to overcome the challenges?
- What will I do differently next time if I do not get the desired results I was seeking?

After My Assignments Are Completed

- Did I pack the completed items that I'll need for class the next day?
- Did I check my home learning to see if I have my name, date, and class number on it?
- Did I hand in any important notes for the teacher as I reflected on the project?
- Did I put my lunch, backpack, and other personal belongings in one place so they will be easy to find and allow me to exit home in a timely fashion?

Home learning reflection sheet

1. What was my overall reaction to the home learning assigment?

2. What strategies seemed to work best?

3. What strategies would I revise?

4. After feedback from the teachers, I will

   Keep:

   Change:

✓ **Self-Regulated Learning Checklist**

Phase One: Pre-action

- Motivation for learning: Why am I doing this activity?
- Short-Term Goals: What do I expect to accomplish in one session?
  Long-Term Goals: What is the due date for the final product?
  Time Management: What breaks am I planning?
- Who can help? Who can I turn to for help?

  Problems that may arise: How will I address challenges that arise?
  Desired Outcome: The end result is?

Phase Two: Monitor

Step 1: Taking in new information
What are two strategies that will allow me to understand new information most effectively?

1. _____

2. _____

Step 2: Organizing information effectively. After I take in new information, how will I organize it?
What are two strategies that will allow me to organize information most effectively?

1. _____

2. _____

Step 3: Understanding/Studying information.
Now that I have collected and organized information, how will it help me?
What are two strategies that will allow me to understand or actively study the information most effectively?

1. _____

2. _____

Phase Three: Self-Reflection

- How do I know if my goals were realistically set?
- Was I satisfied with my end result using the self-regulated principles? If so, what will I do again? If not, why not?
- If I was satisfied with how the task was completed, what will I do again?

As I reflect, I . . .

Things I would continue to do:

Performance: Forethought Phase One

Things I would change:

✓ **Self-Regulation Checklist for Home Learning**

Next steps: I will (Fill in the blanks with yes or no)
  As I reflect, next time I will

1. *I will* _____

2. *I will* _____

3. *I will* _____

✓ **Math Test: Student Studying Checklist**

Before Studying

- Have I mapped out a study schedule for the days leading up to the test?
- Have I planned distributed practice prior to the test and massed practice the day before the test?
- Do I have a quiet, distraction-free environment to study in?
- Do I have access to the necessary math tools? (calculator, ruler, etc.)
- Do I have access to all my unit notes and quizzes for reference?
- Will I use rubrics and exemplars to determine standards?

During Studying

- What is the important information to study? Why do I think it is important?

- Have I reached out to peers with questions on concepts I do not understand?
- Do I take a break when needed?
- Have I rewritten and solved questions from unit quizzes that I had gotten incorrect?
- Do I understand "process" such that if I am given an answer I will be able to explain the steps in solving the problem?

After Studying

- Did I do a good job staying on task? If not, what distractions did I encounter that I need to address next time I study?
- Did I give myself enough time to study or will I have to plan for more time?
- What strategy was most helpful during the process?
- What can I do differently next time to improve my studying?
- Did the material make sense?
- Did the material have meaning?

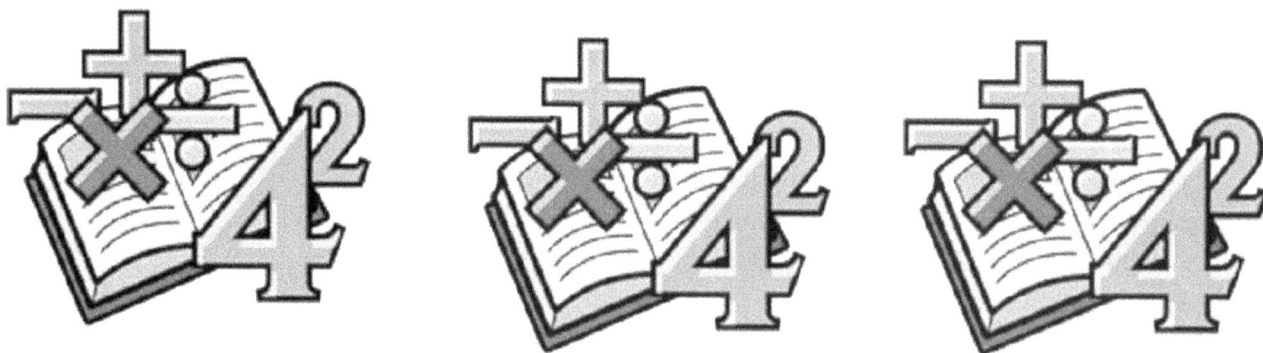

Figure 1.5 Mathematics.

After I received my grade, what study skills will I change?

Change:

Keep:

✓ **Strategies for Students**

When Doing My Homework, I will:

- Pick a good time to do my homework, when I feel rested and alert, not when I am tired.
- Pick a good location to do my homework. Maybe a room with minimal distractions.
- Review my calendar of deadlines. I choose homework assignments that are due first.
- Plan more time for assignments that I feel are more challenging than homework that I find easier for me.
- Use resources when I need additional information. I can search the internet, library, or seek assistance from adults or peers.
- I will try to remember the information my teacher covered in class so I can answer questions correctly.
- When learning new information I will make connections to information I already know.
- I will schedule small breaks after I attend to my homework for a designated amount of time to allow my brain to recharge.
- I will picture myself handing in an incomplete assignment to my teacher the next day when I feel that I do not want to complete my homework assignment.

Reflection

- I will use the feedback from the teacher to improve for the next assignment.

When Studying for a Test, I Will:

- Try to come up with questions that I believe will be found on the test.
- Copy my notes to try to remember the material being covered.
- Make a chart of important words and information to review.
- Create study cards / index cards for me to review at later times in the day.
- Outline/highlight important information and details from the text.
- Teach the information to someone else to help me process the information.
- Ask myself questions on the material to ensure I am internalizing the information.
- Use mnemonic devices to help me memorize facts.
- Consider joining a study group in the library to collaborate with my peers.
- Think of the grade I am trying to achieve on my report card.

THE LEARNER'S BRAIN MODEL

Summary of the Chapter

Activities and worksheets were provided for adults to promote long-term learning and for student self-regulation.

Self-Regulation

The most important skill that educators can develop in students is the ability to control aspects of their learning. Student self-regulation is one way to control aspects of their learning and to take ownership. Without this ability, the students are teacher dependent and not self-dependent.

A self-dependent student has the ability to monitor and control her own behavior, emotions, or thoughts, and to be able to alter them based on the demands of the situation. It includes the abilities to inhibit reactive initial responses, to resist interference from irrelevant stimulation, and to persist with relevant tasks to achieve a goal.

Strategies for Self-Regulation

This chapter has examples of self-regulated checklists and strategies for students to use, including:

Study strategies for students
Home-learning checklists
How to keep binders organized
Self-regulation for home learning

Conclusion

Research suggests that aspects of teaching effectiveness make the difference in how students perform. Successful teachers tend to be those who employ a range of teaching strategies and interactive styles to meet the needs of their learners. These effective teachers utilize different instructional goals, topics, and methods. Research further demonstrates that teachers' abilities to structure material, ask higher-order questions, use student ideas, and probe student comments have also been found to be important variables in what students learn.

More importantly, the learner has to be involved in the process and has to become a self- regulated learner so she is not teacher or school dependent but self-dependent.

REFERENCES

Bloom, B. S. (1956). *Taxonomy of Educational Objectives: The Classification of Educational Goals, Handbook 1: Cognitive Domain*. New York: David McKay.

Bookheimer, S.Y., Zeffiro, T.A., Blaxton, T.A., Gaillard, P.W., and Theodore, W.H. (2000) Activation of language cortex with automatic speech tasks *Neurology*, 55(8): 1151-1157.

Bush, G. (1990). Presidential Proclamation 6158. (Library of Congress), available at http://leweb.loc.gov/loc/brain/proclaim.html

Cowley, G., and Underwood, A. (1998, June 15). Memory. *Newsweek*, *131*(24).

Dewey, John. (1895). The Theory of Emotion, (1): Emotional Attitudes. *Psychological Review*, 1: 553–569.

Dewey, John. (1896). The Reflex Arc Concept in Psychology. *Psychological Review*, 3.

Dewey, John. (1902). *The Child and the Curriculum*. Chicago: University of Chicago Press.

Dewey, John. (1902) The School and Society.

Dewey, John. (1910). *How We Think*. Lexington, MA: D. C. Heath.

Dewey, John. (1915). *Schools of Tomorrow*. New York: Dutton Press.

Dewey, John. (1916). The Relationship of Thought and Its Subject Matter, chapter 2 in *Essays in Experimental Logic*. Chicago: University of Chicago Press.

Dewey, John. (1933). *How We Think: A Restatement of the Relation of Reflective Thinking of the Educative Process*. Boston: D. C. Heath.

Dewey, John. (1938). *Experience and Education*. New York: Collier Books.

Diamond, M., and Hopson, J. (1998). Magic trees of the mind: How to nurture your child's intelligence, creativity and healthy emotions from birth through adolescence. New York: Penguin Putnam.

Ebbinghaus, Hermann. (1885). *Memory: A Contribution to Experimental Psychology* (Henry A. Ruger and Clara E. Bussenino, Trans., 1913). New York: Teachers College Press, Columbia University.

Holloway, John. (2000, November). How does the brain learn science? *Educational Leadership*, *58*(3).

Hunter, M. (1979, October). Teaching is decision making. *Educational Leadership*.

Hunter, M. (1982). *Mastery Teaching*. El Segundo, CA: TIP Publications.

Huttenlocher, P. R., and Dabholkan, A. S. (1997). Regional differences in synaptogenesis in human cerebral cortex. *Journal of Comparative Neurology*, *387*.

Jensen, Eric. (1998). How Julie's brain learns. *Educational Leadership*, *51*(3).

Krug, Mark. (1972) *What Will Be Taught: The Next Decade*. Itasca, IL: F. E. Peacock.

Lepore, F. (2001, January 1). Dissecting genius: Einstein's brain and the search for the neural basis of intellect. New York: Dana Foundation.

Praxis. (1995). Paper presented at the Annual Meeting of the American Education Research Association, San Francisco, CA, April 18–22.

Ramey, C. T., and Ramey, S. L. (1996, February). At risk does not mean doomed. Paper presented at a meeting of the American Association of Science. National Health/Education Consortium Occasional Paper #4.

Sousa, David. (2000). *How the Brain Learns*. Thousand Oaks, CA: Corwin Press.

Sousa, David. (2001). *How the Brain Learns* (2nd ed.). Thousand Oaks, CA: Corwin Press.

Sousa, David. (2001). *How the Special Needs Brain Learns*. Thousand Oaks, CA: Corwin Press.

Wolfe, Pat. (1999). Revisiting effective teaching. *Educational Leadership*, *56*(3), 61-64.

Wolfe, Patricia. (2001). *Brain Matters: Translating Research into Classroom Practice*. Alexandria, VA: Association for Supervision and Curriculum Development.

The Knowing

Planning and Establishing for the Instructional Domain

FOCUS OF THE CHAPTER

The chapter begins unpacking the Learner's Brain Model. Please refer to the text *Setting the Stage: Delivering the Plan by Using the Learner's Brain Model* by Dr. Mario C. Barbiere for more information.

The first step of the model is planning/readiness and establishing the learning domain. The role of climate, environment, emotional security, mood, and classroom management are parts of the Learner's Brain Model that will be addressed.

INTRODUCTION

This chapter will define the following areas of lesson design for the Learner's Brain Model: Planning, Instruction, Establishing the Domain, Developing the Essential Question, Planning the Student Learning Target (Objective), and assessing the target via a teacher assessment of learning known as a "Demonstration of Student Learning," which is referred to throughout this book as a DSL.

PROBING QUESTIONS

As a teacher, parent, or administrator, there are questions that should be addressed:

1. How does what I want my scholars to know impact my lesson planning?
2. How will I know learning occurred?
3. What are strategies students can use to self-regulate their learning during this phase?

LESSON DESIGN FOR THE LEARNER'S BRAIN MODEL: THE PLANNING STAGE

The first phase of instruction is the planning stage. This stage is specifically geared toward analyzing the data from the previous lesson as well as the information from the formative assessments and checks for understanding that were conducted. The data will determine what should be taught. It involves learning what needs to be done and how instruction should be implemented and delivered.

> **Disposition: An effective lesson requires pre-planning so transitions are smooth, student problems are anticipated, and varied strategies are planned to address the anticipated problems.**

Lesson Design: The Planning Stage

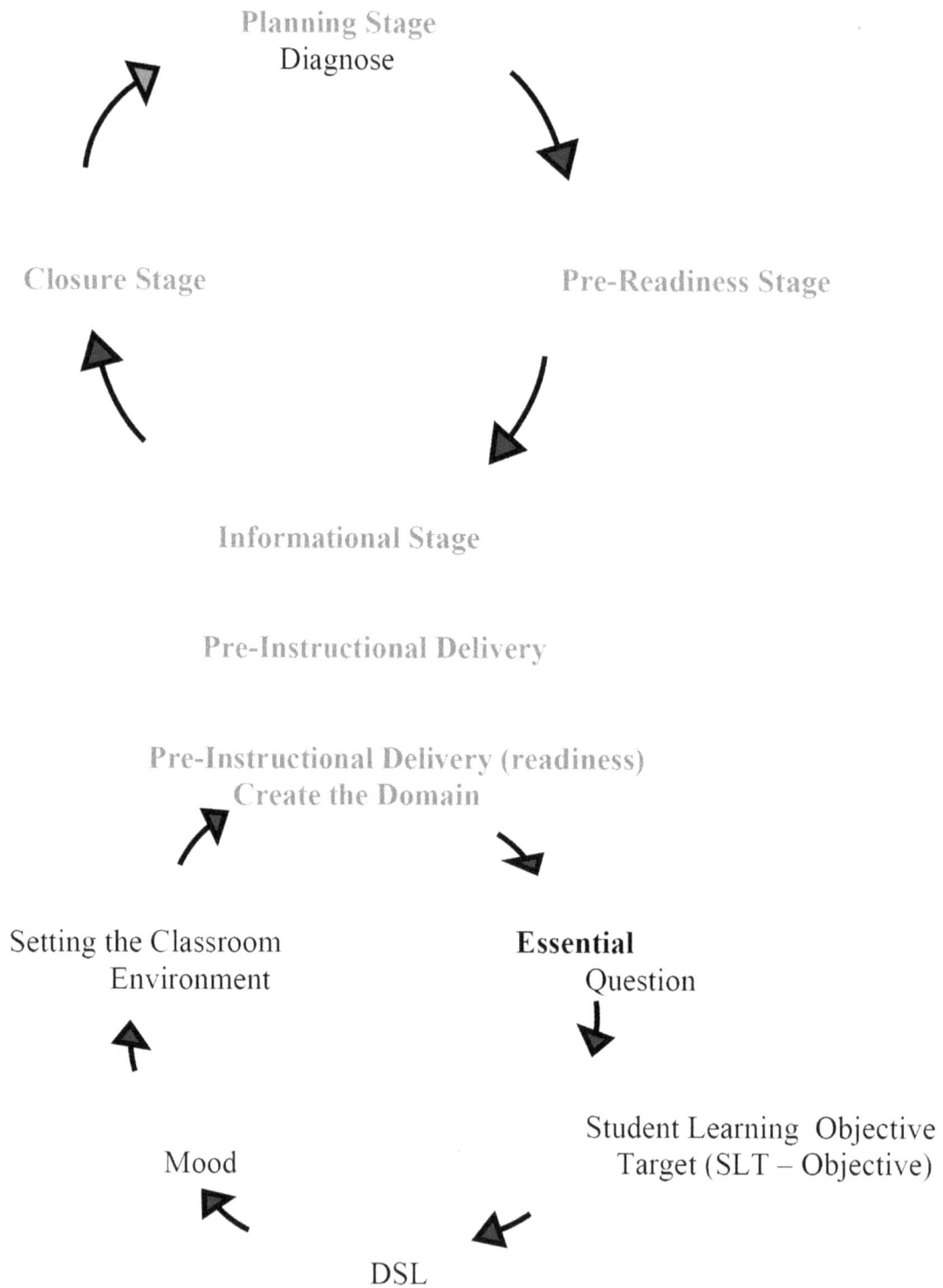

Planning Stage
Diagnose

Closure Stage

Pre-Readiness Stage

Informational Stage

Pre-Instructional Delivery

Pre-Instructional Delivery (readiness)
Create the Domain

Setting the Classroom
Environment

Essential
Question

Student Learning Objective
Target (SLT – Objective)

Mood

DSL

Figure 2.1 Lesson design: The planning stage.

Draw a schema for your Pre-Instructional Delivery.

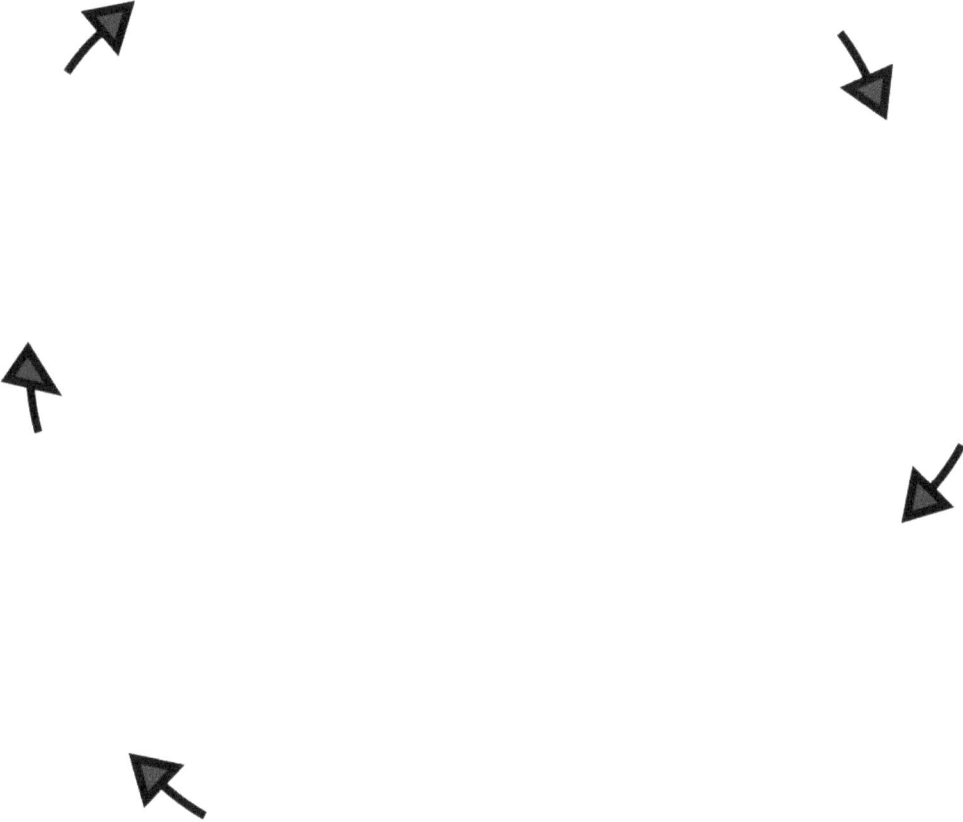

Figure 2.2 A schema for your pre-instructional delivery

Reflection

Activity: Compare and Contrast

Your schema	Learner's Brain Model	Findings

Reflection:

_____

_____

_____

_____

_____

Figure 2.3 Compare and contrast.

REFLECTIVE QUESTIONS FOR SETTING INSTRUCTIONAL OUTCOMES

> **Focus: The teacher establishes instructional outcomes based on what students will be expected to learn and not activities. The outcomes reflect various types of learning and various assessments used and are student friendly.**

- What verbs from Bloom's Revised Taxonomy will I use in planning the Student Learning Target?
- How will the Student Learning Target be conveyed to the student?
- How will I promote high-level learning?
- Is my Student Learning Target clear and stated in terms of student learning rather than student activity?
- How will the instructional delivery be aligned to the Student Learning Target?
- Is the lesson balanced among different types of learning styles?
- Is the Student Learning Target appropriate to the diverse students, i.e., age and developmental level, prior skills and knowledge, and interests and backgrounds?
- Does the Student Learning Target promote cognitive rigor?
- Does the Student Learning Target reflect what will be taught as a skill or concept and not an activity?
- Is my Demonstration of Student Learning going to measure the Student Learning Target?

> **Look For: The SLT are challenging and employ higher cognitive levels. The DSLs used to assess are differentiated and specific to the SLT using higher-level verbs.**

REFLECTIVE QUESTIONS FOR FINALIZING COHERENT INSTRUCTION

> **Focus: The teacher's planning reflects knowledge of content, students, and available resources. Instruction is designed to cognitively engage students. Instructional groups organized to support differentiated student learning are flexible and skills based. Outcomes measure what was taught and are not activities.**

- How will the instructional outcomes, activities, materials, methods, and the grouping of students be aligned?
- Is there a logical sequence of activities planned?
- Was there a clearly recognizable structure to the lesson?
- How will the instructional activities be designed? Specifically, "What will the student *do* in order to learn X?" (Direct instruction, work in small groups to solve a problem, or engage in a project then participate in class discussions?)
- How will the lesson be designed to cognitively challenge students so they can have the opportunity to develop their own understanding?
- Will there be an opportunity for students to engage in reflection and closure?
- What data will be used to develop the lessons?
- Will additional activities be planned for students who excel during the lesson?

> **Look For: A structured lesson plan in which resources are varied, activities require high-level thinking, and grouping based on student abilities or skill development.**

DESIGNING STUDENT ASSESSMENTS

> **Focus: The focus is on assessment of learning. Did the students achieve the learning targets? Are the assessments adapted to standards? Will the lesson be adapted as needed based on the assessments done throughout the lesson?**

- How will checks for understanding be used as assessments *of* learning (to determine if students have achieved the instructional outcomes established through the planning process)?
- Will teachers who work with the same students share data?
- Are assessments *for* learning planned (assessment that provides both the teacher and student with valuable information to guide future learning, typically undertaken by teachers on their own in response to their individual groups of students)?
- Will students engage in self-regulated learning using a scoring system or a rubric for evaluating their work?
- Is there a plan for students to participate in the designing of assessments?
- Will students develop or contribute test or quiz questions?

> **Look For: Lesson plans include assessments congruent with instructional outcomes. Assessments are planned throughout lesson to inform instructional delivery and students know how they will be assessed. Provisions are made for students with learning or reading concerns. Students are able to self-regulate their learning with the use of rubrics, exemplars, or feedback.**

Brain Research: The Essential Question (EQ) enables the learner's brain to search for complete-

ness. In essence, the brain is looking for a pattern between the lesson and the Essential Question to make a "visual connection." This will promote "visual thinking."

SRL: This practice of seeking completeness begins self-regulated learning by informing the student of the daily Student Learning Target (SLT) and how it relates to the big picture (EQ). The students will be able to monitor and modulate their learning.

What: The Essential Question is the "big idea" or concept. The Student Learning Target (Objective) addresses how the long term concept will be achieved.

Why: *The Essential Question* encourages the student to consider the "big idea" so the student can plan a path or direction in their thinking to achieve the goal. Understanding that there is an array of potential answers, to meet the objective knowing the desired result will be helpful to frame the student's thinking during the lesson.

Where: Posting or stating an essential question prior to the lesson and after the Readiness Set, is consistent with the brain's processing of visual information in a holistic manner.

WRITING THE STUDENT LEARNING TARGET (OBJECTIVE)

Brain Research: In essence, the brain is looking for a visual pattern on how everything is connected to the end goal. This is known as "visual thinking or visual mapping."

Student Learning Target (Objective): The Student Learning Target (Objective) enables the student's brain to understand the purpose of the lesson and what the student will be learning.

SRL: The practice of posting the Student Learning Target (SLT) and Essential Question helps the student begin the process of self-regulation.

	Performance: Forethought Phase 1
	Do I know the goal/objective of the assignment?
	Am I accomplishing the goal?
	Have I broken down the assignment into achievable parts?
	Do I know what type of environment I need to do my best work?
	Do I know what questions to ask myself while working?
	Do I know how to motivate myself?
	Performance: Monitor and Regulate Phase 2
	Do I know the goal/objective of the assignment?
	Am I accomplishing the goal?
	Have I broken down the assignment into achievable parts?
	Is the environment working for me to do my best work?
	Do I know what questions to ask myself while working?
	Do I know how to motivate myself?
	Reflection-Phase 3
	Did I re-read the instructions and check my work?
	Did I use my time efficiently?
	Did I place my finished work in my "Return to School" folder?
	Did I reward myself? ☺
	Did I get feedback from my teacher, parents, or peers?

Next steps: I will (Fill in the blanks)

1. I will _____

2. I will _____

3. I will _____

4. I will _____

Reflection:

HOW IS A STUDENT LEARNING TARGET (OBJECTIVE) DEVELOPED?

The student objective has two components to it. One part is Cognition (some may know it as behavior), which is what the student is expected to learn.

The second part to the student objective is Calibration (measurement) and that is how the learning will be measured. The Demonstration of Student Learning (DSL) is the vehicle for calibration (the measurement that will enable the teacher to calibrate her teaching). The two components are like bookends as the objective identifies the desired student cognition and the Demonstration of Student Learning is the measurement of the learning. In between the two bookends is the instructional delivery (condition) and student self-regulation. For students, the teacher must write a student friendly objective of what the student will be learning and a Demonstration of the Student Learning that informs the student how they will be assessed. The information from the Demonstration of Student Learning will help the teacher calibrate her lesson and future lessons.

It is important to note that there is a third component called "condition." The Condition part of the objective is the instructional delivery to be used by the teacher and is valuable for an administrator. The administrator will see the instructional strategies a teacher plans to use and has used over the course of the year. The administrator will be able to see the teacher's variety of execution used in instructional delivery.

For the student, a student friendly objective is important because it is the cognition (what the student will learn) and calibration (assessment of how the student will demonstrate knowledge) that is important.

The three components of a Student Learning Target (objective)—cognition, condition, and calibration—are necessary for administrators. The two parts, cognition and calibration, are necessary for the student.

When writing an objective, the task is to focus on student learning and not on developing an objective written for the administrator. The teacher should ask: What cognition am I seeking and what do I expect the student to know and do? If those questions are to be considered, the teacher will write the Student Learning Target as: "I will be able to do . . . Once that aspect of the SLT (objective) is developed, the teacher will be able to determine how the student will demonstrate their knowledge. The Demonstration of Student Learning (DSL) can be written as "I will" statement: I will be able to demonstrate, explain, justify, or any other high-level verb that will promote student metacognition.

Model for Writing Student Learning Targets (Objectives)

INTRODUCTION

- Objectives have three distinct components: Cognition, Condition, and Calibration for administrators. Student objectives have two components: Cognition and Calibration.

COGNITION (DESIRED STUDENT LEARNING)

- Describes learner capability. Use action verbs when developing the behavior.
- Must be observable and measurable (you will define the measurement elsewhere).
- It should be a skill tied to a standard and not an activity.
- The "behavior" can include demonstration of knowledge or skills in any of the domains of learning: factual, conceptual, procedural, or metacognitive.
- Example: I will be able to write a report . . . (factual)
- Example: I will be able to classify, interpret, show . . . (conceptual)
- Example: I can justify, illustrate, infer . . . (procedural)

- Example: I can create . . . (metacognitive)
- Cognitive domains
  - Cognitive domain (low level, entry level)
    - Emphasizes remembering or reproducing something that has presumably been learned. Can involve making a list, highlighting, describing, locating information.
    - Addresses what a learner should know, understand, comprehend, solve, spell, critique, etc., at a level of recall, locating, describing, or selecting from a list. This process is at a recognition level (getting background information of facts and data) for the learner's brain.
  - Conceptual domain
    - Emphasizes the student's ability to demonstrate, explain information, give examples to show understanding, draw a representation, make conclusions based on the information, or explain an idea.
    - This domain is concerned with the student showing understanding of the big picture or the concept of the skill. Hence the ability to build, organize, or solve a problem.
  - Procedural domain
    - The ability of the learner to apply the concepts learned.
    - The learner will be able to make inferences, apply information to solve problems, critique, justify statements based on facts or evidence, or prove mathematical problems.
  - Metacognitive domain
    - Emphasizes learner's skill and ability to design, create, compose, or improve a product.
    - Emphasizes how a learner tests theories, constructs new creative solutions, or generates new ideas.

CONDITION (INSTRUCTIONAL DELIVERY)

- How the teacher will deliver the lesson. This fact is important for administrators so they can see the various teaching techniques employed by a teacher.
- "After" and "given" are usually the "target words" that normally precede the condition.
- Example: Given (target word for condition) a short personal narrative, I will cite three details from the text to analyze how a significant incident in the narrator's life provokes a decision and reveals aspects of his/her character.
- Example: Given selected works of William Shakespeare, I will be able to . . .
- Example: After a discussion about the following environment: 10 p.m., snowing, temperature 0 degrees C, I will . . . (The "I will" begins the behavior part of the objective.)

CALIBRATION (MEASUREMENT OF PERFORMANCE)

- States the standard for acceptable measurement performance (time, accuracy, proportion, quality, etc.)
- DSL is tied to the objective as it is a measurement of the objective.
- Example of accepted performance: . . . without error.
- Example of expected performance: . . . 9 out of 10 times; receiving a three on a four-point rubric.
- Review the following weak and strong examples of Student Learning Targets (Objectives).

In your own words:

Cognition is	My examples
Condition is	My examples
Calibration is	My examples

WHAT IS A DEMONSTRATION OF STUDENT LEARNING (DSL)?

What: A Demonstration of Student Learning (DSL) is an activity or product in which a student demonstrates that she has learned the lesson and can demonstrate mastery of the objective by producing a product, a performance, or a written task. DSLs can be done at the end of a daily lesson or the end of a longer two-day lesson.

Why: One phase of self-regulation is student motivation and student monitoring. The purpose of the DSL is for students to know what the teacher's expectation is for the student to demonstrate their learning.

Where: Posted under the Student Learning Target (Objective), the students will know what they are learning (Student Learning Target) and how they will be held accountable (Demonstration of Student Learning).

Brain Research: The Demonstration of Student Learning and the Student Learning Target enables the learner to see completeness. The brain seeks completeness in order for information to be processed. Where there is no completeness, the brain will attempt to fill in the completeness as in optical illusions. Seeking completeness is a task of the brain. Additionally, self-efficacy is the extent or strength of one's belief in one's own ability to complete tasks and reach goals. One must know what they are in order to work toward completing them.

SRL: Demonstration of Student Learning (DSL) is consistent with the monitoring and management stage of self-regulation.

Activity Worksheet

Student Learning Target (Objective)	Weak	*Student Learning Target (Objective)*	Strong
Students will understand			
We will examine how ancient people developed technology			
Complete page 33 in the workbook			
Today you will: be introduced to the new vocabulary words from one of our core novel			

REFLECTION: Characteristics of a strong Student Learning Target (Objective). I notice, I wonder

ACTIVITY for Student Learning targets and Demonstrations of Student Learning

Student Learning Target
(Objective)

Instructional Delivery

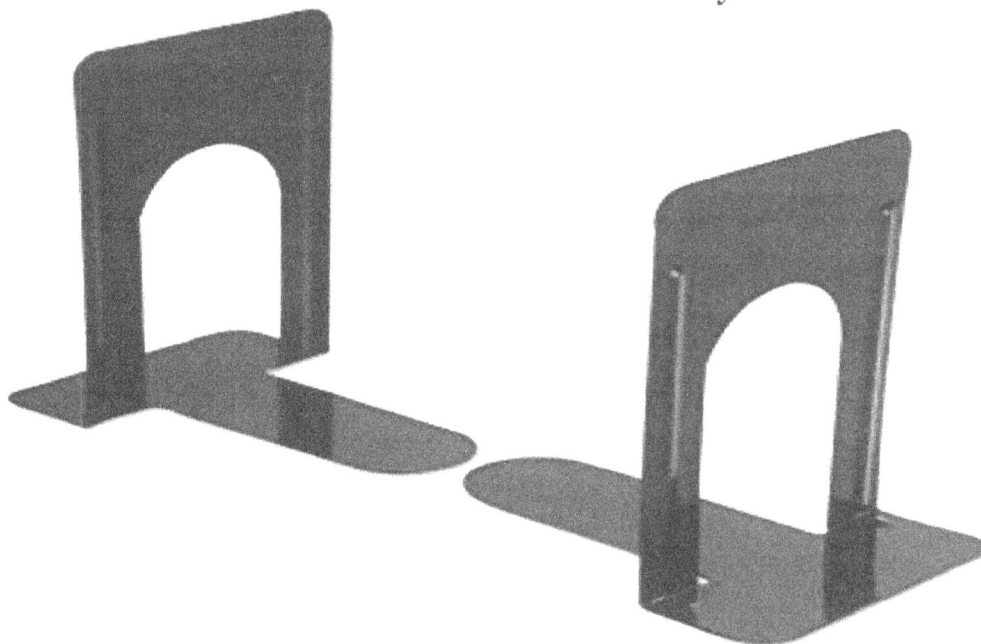

Demonstration of Learning
(DSL)

My Student Learning Target is:

The Demonstration of Student Learning is:

The instructional activities I would use are:"

Reminder: A well-crafted DSL will include the following.

1. The posted DSL will help the student recognize what is expected of them and will help the student to frame the teaching relative to teacher expectation. Knowing this, the student can start the process of internalizing information relative to what is being assessed.
2. The DSL should include evidence that the skill has been met.
3. The DSL should capture the essence of what the teacher taught and be presented by the student either verbally or written.
4. The DSL should be specific to the objective.

The Demonstration of Student Learning (DSL)

Exercise of Effective Assessment of Learning Targets (Demonstration of Student Learning) (DSL).

Review the following weak and strong examples of Demonstration of Student Learning.

Weak Assessment of Demonstration of Student Learning (DSL)	Strong Assessment of Demonstration of Student Learning (DSL)
Students will complete a worksheet	
Students will correctly get 3 out of 6 examples correct	
Student will do the odd problems on a worksheet	
Students will submit an exit ticket at the end of the lesson	
Students will find the main idea from the article they were given	

REFLECTION: Characteristics of a strong Demonstration of Student Learning DSL))

Activity: Bring a Student Learning Target and its Demonstration of Student Learning. Using the information below, assess your Demonstration of Student Learning.

My Student Learning Target:

My Demonstration of Student Learning:

The DSL should tie directly into the lesson objective and the guaranteed curriculum.

1. The DSL can usually be accomplished in a short period of time, from 5 to 10 minutes.
2. The DSL is measurable.
3. The DSL requires students to demonstrate or perform what they have learned.
4. The DSL varies from day to day.
5. The DSL is understandable to students and parents.
6. The DSL is not a check for understanding.
7. The DSL is done after the lesson is taught.
8. Multiple DSLs can be used via the use of multiple intelligences.

Any changes to my DSL? If so, write it below. If not, what is your assessment?

My assessment:

Fact Sheet

The relationship between Revised Bloom's Taxonomy (RBT) and the Relationship to Webb's Depth of Knowledge (DOK) when developing Student Learning Targets

I. Background: The three Cs of objective construction

1. Constructing objectives involves using three parts: Cognition (student learning), Condition (teacher methodology, and Calibration (measurement).
2. Cognition: what the student is expected to do.
3. Condition: what the teacher will do and/or how the teacher will do it. This is usually prefaced by the target word after or given. For example, after a discussion about the Civil War, I will be able to identify key battles and why the battles were significant.
4. Calibration (measurement): the assessment of the learning to determine if the student has learned the skill or concept of the objective. The teacher calibrates the future lessons based on the information received.
5. The use of the verbs and the nouns in the Student Learning Target is extremely important as they promote the level of cognition desired by the teacher.

Student Objective (two parts) Cognition   +   Calibration: DSL
Cognition is what the student will learn

measurement of what was taught or an assessment of the student learning. The student demonstrates knowledge and the teacher collects the data to plan future lessons

II. Deconstructing the Student Friendly Objective

1. The purpose of the Student Learning Target (SLT-objective) is to inform the student of what is expected so the student can begin the process of self-regulation. (This is the beginning of the process and it is referred to as Forethought).
2. The objective is for the student to know what they will be learning. The student will know how she will be assessed by the teacher or a peer on what was taught to determine if she learned the concept.
3. Example of an objective: I will be able to analyze and explain the difference between the form of government in Switzerland (confederation), United States (federal), and China (unitary).
4. Deconstructing the objective noted above
   a. Who: I (the learner)
   b. What: distinguishing by analyzing then justifying the three types of systems

c. How: by comparing, contrasting, analyzing, and justifying the types of systems. In the teacher's plan book, the teacher will plan for differentiation of the groups. For math, the process of "Gradual Release" involves you do, we do, and I do.

III. Deconstructing the verbs and nouns in the objective

1. The verb
   a. The verb in the objective drives the cognitive process the student will use. Teachers should be mindful of this fact and use verbs that promote metacognition.
   b. Why using the term Cognition as opposed to Behavior? When the term "behavior" is used, people will think of the action as the process of behaviorism, i.e., instrumental conditioning, stimulus response, or teaching through manipulatives or teacher-directed instruction. With a behaviorism mindset, students are being "conditioned"—conditional learning prompted by rewards. In essence the student is not regulating their own learning but being lead or "trained" to think in a certain way.
   c. If one changes the word "behavior" to cognition (or the cognitive process) then we focus on the student learning as opposed to a stimulus response, condition learning. Using higher-level verbs also promotes a higher level of cognition: metacognition.
   d. Using the term behavior implies the objective is a means to an end or an activity the student will be doing so as to be "conditioned."
   e. Another reason for substituting the term cognition is that it implies an end product of what the teacher wants the students to learn.
   f. Asking the simple question "what do we want the student to learn?" will distinguish between an activity or a cognitive learning outcome. Students will learn to solve equa-

tions into unknowns. Students will learn to solve equations with two unknowns using three different methods, is a cognitive task.
   g. An example for reading is: Reading an article is an activity while determining the point of view using evidence from an article is a cognitive task promoted by the objective.
   h. *Summary: The verb in the objective is the driver for the cognition that the student must do, not the activity a student will be doing.*
2. The noun
   a. The noun of the Student Learning Target (objective) is the knowledge that the student will be using. The levels, according to Bloom, move from remembering factual knowledge to conceptual knowledge, which is putting the facts together to understand concepts. After the concepts are learned and practiced, they become procedural. The highest level is creating or metacognition. The task is to have the student move from isolated individual facts to concepts (big picture) and being able to understand the integration of information.
   b. *The noun of the Student Learning Target (objective) is the content that the student is expected to know.*

IV. Webb's Depth of Knowledge (DOK) is a vehicle to assess curriculum

1. Webb's Depth of Knowledge (DOK) was developed in 1997 as a process and criteria for systematically analyzing the alignment between standards and standardized assessments. It is also a means to review curriculum alignment.
2. The purpose of the DOK is to analyze the cognition expectations demanded by standards, curriculum activities, and assessment task as defined by Webb (1997).
3. *DOK background.* There are four levels and in the Depth of Knowledge schema, and the

four levels reflect a different level of cognitive expectations required to complete the task. The four levels are:

a. *Level I: Recall and Reproduction level for factual knowledge.* In this model the teacher would be doing most of the talking during the instructional period by asking students to tell, remember, list, recall, identify key words, or make a timeline. In this scenario, the teacher is telling students facts and information, using who, what, where, when, and how types of questions to get the student to recall facts and/or be able to develop basic knowledge about the critical attributes of what she is teaching.

For example, if the teacher is teaching about three different systems of government, the student has to know specific details about each type of government. The verbs used to develop this knowledge would be at the remembering and understanding level of Revised Bloom's Taxonomy unless the teacher had students compare and contrast the different systems. That activity would involve analysis, evaluation, and synthesis of information.

b. *Level II: Skills and Concepts. In this level, the student is going beyond recalling facts to a more analytical approach of thinking.* In this level, the student is taking the facts, interpreting the facts, then applying them. The student at this level is applying the factual skills into concepts in an integrated manner. The teacher can help with the process by asking the student to calculate or construct the knowledge so as to apply the facts. Verbs suggested for applying knowledge would cause a learner to analyze, interpret, and explain factual information. Other verbs to promote application of knowledge would include analyze, categorize, integrate, compare, contrast, and differentiate.

c. *Level III: Short-Term Strategic Thinking. In this level the student will be analyzing and evaluating the concepts to be able to explain a concept with supporting evidence.* A teacher may have the student create a spreadsheet, chart, report, do a podcast, or conduct an investigation to promote strategic thinking. The teacher's role would be to ask probing questions, ask students to classify data, clarify or evaluate their thinking. Students are encouraged to extend their thinking beyond the facts. The student is challenged to justify their reasoning with facts and not just an opinion.

Students can demonstrate their learning at the strategic level by using Venn diagrams to show relationships, conduct an investigation, develop a rubric, develop research questions or a hypothesis to test, or propose a solution to a problem. Verbs from the analyzing level include analyze, apply, produce, show, solve, or use. The goal is to encourage the learner to analyze information to evaluate and apply strategic thinking.

d. *Level IV: Extended Thinking.* This level uses higher-order thinking and is promoted by synthesizing information. It involves creative solutions to problems. The teacher is facilitating evaluation, reflection, and analysis to promote the student to design, create, modify, or suggest new iterations of the product. Higher-level verbs like evaluate and create would promote extended thinking.

V. Relationship of Revised Bloom's Taxonomy to Webb's Depth of Knowledge

In the previous example, a sample objective was provided. Let's dissect that example.

I will be able to analyze and justify the difference between the form of government in Switzerland (confederation), United States (federal), and China (unitary system).

A breakdown is below.

Verbs	Nouns
Analyze and justify	Confederate, federal, unitary systems
The learner will be comparing, contrasting or collecting evidence and data about the three systems to justify their answer	The student will be researching systems to analyze how they are the same or different so as to make comparisons between the three systems.
Revised Bloom's Taxonomy – Level 4: analyze and justify	DOK - Level 3

Activity
Select an objective and rate the verb in the objective using Revised Bloom's Taxonomy. Look at the nouns in the objective and rank the nouns (like the example.) What do you notice?

I noticed:

After you do that activity, change the verb to a different level, and using the same noun, think about what activities one would have to do to achieve the objective.

Verb	Noun
(list the verb)	(list the noun)
Write	Think about the activities needed to meet the objective
Revised Bloom's Taxonomy – Level	DOK - Level

New Sample by changing the verb

(list the verb)	
Rewrite the objective using a different verb	Think about activities needed to meet the new objective
Revised Bloom's Taxonomy – Level	DOK - Level

CRITICAL CONSIDERATIONS FOR THE TEACHER

Teacher's role: the instructional implications are:

1. Knowing where the student is relative to their prior knowledge. Knowing the student's prior knowledge becomes a starting point for the lesson.
2. Determining what information is needed in the instructional delivery to provide critical facts and information so the students can use the facts to solve problems.
3. Verbs that teachers use in developing the objectives for students impacted cognition that the student will be performing.
4. Nouns in the objective address content knowledge.
5. Student performance can be rated using the Depth of Knowledge chart.
6. Higher level of Revised Bloom's Taxonomy will yield a higher level of cognition on the Depth of Knowledge.
7. Cognitive levels move from factual (knowing facts and information), conceptual (understanding concepts and "big pictures"), procedural (applying concepts) to metacognition (thinking about one's thinking).

Your reactions:

Checklist for the development of Student Learning Target (objective) and Demonstration of Student Learning (DSL)

	Objective		Indicators	Considerations/Tasks
Alignment	- Objective ties to Essential Question - Objective aligns Common Core - Objective addresses a skill to be assessed by a CRT, curriculum benchmark or curriculum map Aligns to District Curriculum	☐ ☐ ☐ ☐ ☐	- High-level verbs used - Objective and DSL linked and aligned to standards - Objective is an expectation for skill development and not an activity	- Are Common Core standards "unpacked" in the development of the objective? - Does the objective lead to deeper understanding of the concept? - What is the desired student outcome?
Behavior	- Objective is written using "I" - Objective stresses a student outcome and is not an activity - Lower levels of RBT used to promote factual knowledge which will lead to application (developmental level of skill) - Higher-level verbs used to promote metacognition - Content and process linked and lead to the development of "dispositions"	☐ ☐ ☐ ☐ ☐	- Begins with "I can, I will" - Clear, specific, measurable so students know what to do - RBT used to develop factual knowledge and base for developing application - Higher-level verbs used in the assessment of the skill - Is the skill needed for the development of a disposition?	- Objective and DSL written in student friendly terms and appropriate for the age/grade level to promote Self-Regulated Learning - Factual knowledge necessary to develop creative thinking (Willingham, 2011) to develop skill base for later use - Assessment (DSL) requires analysis, evaluation, or creation to show mastery - "Disposition," i.e., student learns how to read to develop a desire to read
Condition	- Various strategies planned to deliver the lesson - Delivery of the lesson addresses various student modalities - Technology planned to enhance lesson - Delivery will promote varied grouping practices (large to small groups)	☐ ☐ ☐ ☐	- Instructional strategies based on student needs. - Variety of learning styles used throughout the lesson - Technology planned for teacher and student use - An outcome of the delivery will lead to flexible grouping	- Varied modalities planned throughout the year - Students will be able to work at their own pace and self-manage their time - Technology available for student use and differentiation of lesson - Flexible grouping or use of anchor activities for students who finish early
DSL/Measurement	- Clear connection to objective - High level of Bloom's Taxonomy verbs used to assess the learning - Written in student friendly terms - Measurable—assesses what was taught - Multiple measures of assessment can be used to show mastery - Assessment can be linked to other disciplines - DSL will allow student to create other measures of assessment - DSL will lead to "dispositions"	☐ ☐ ☐ ☐ ☐ ☐ ☐	- Objective/DSL congruent - RBT used with emphasis on analyze, evaluate, or create - Students can articulate DSL - Measurement based on rubric or standards - Opportunity for the use of some multiple intelligences - Interdisciplinary approach used for the activities planned - Student will be able to use multiple measures - DSL mastery shows knowledge skill	- Based on student application of information using analysis, interpretation, or creativity - "I can or I will show" the teacher - Measurement known to student so student can self-assess throughout lesson - Use of multiple intelligences for product based on student ability - Real-world application promoted to show application of disciplines - Student expands original assessment to develop other assessments - Broader applications are expected
Teacher questions	*- What will the student be learning today?* *- How will I cognitively challenge the student?* *- Do you feel today's lesson has high expectations for your learning?*	*Student expectation*	*- Student products will reflect deeper understanding and application of skills* *- Students will think of other ways to show the teacher they learned today's lesson*	*- Students can self-regulate and monitor throughout the lesson as they know what they are learning and how they will be assessed.* *- Students will use varied assessments to show teacher their depth on knowledge.*

Activity

On the chart below, you are identifying two things. One task is to identify the questions a teacher is asking a student using Revised Bloom's Taxonomy. The first two levels of Revised Bloom's Taxonomy (RBTR) correspond to Webb's Depth of Knowledge (DOK) Quadrant 1; the next level of RBT corresponds to DOK Quadrant 2; the next level of RBT corresponds to DOK Quadrant 3 and the two higher levels of RBT correspond to DOK Quadrant 4. As the teacher asks student #1 a question, 1 is put by the question category. For example, if the teacher says to a student, "Identify what X did in the story," the recorder would put a 1 in the "what" category.

Revised Bloom's Taxonomy   Webb's Depth of Knowledge

Verbs	Instructional Strategies	Model questions	Quadrant 3: PROBING QUESTIONS Promotes STRATEGIC THINKING (DOK LEVEL 3 STRATEGIC)	Quadrant 4: RECONSTRUCT/INSPIRE: Promotes EXTENDED THINKING (DOK LEVEL 4: EXTENDED THINKING)
Compose, construct, design, device predict	Design, create, devise or compose	how would you test, develop a creative solution, invent a new system, process, procedure		
appraise, argue, estimate, criticize, debate, justify, verify	justify, prioritize and rationalize, debate, evaluate	invalid?, Judge the effects, finding errors, defend your point of view, justify your answer, isn't biased, fair or ethical?		
Apply, explain, generalize, judge, organize, produce, show, sketch, solve, use	Apply in the real world, case study, construct a model, explain an idea	Predict what would happen, Tell me how, when, where and why?, Identify the results of ..?, What is the function of...? Choose the best statements that apply....	Quadrant 1: OPEN/CLOSED QUESTIONS. Promotes RECALL (DOK LEVEL 1: RECALL)	Quadrant 2: LEADING QUESTIONS Promotes SKILL/CONCEPTS (DOK LEVEL 2:SKILLS)
analyze, categorize, cause/effect compare, contrast, differentiated	Jigsaw activity, What are the assumptions, relationship, and	Is that fact or opinion, What are the assumptions? What does the author believe?, What is the relationship between..? , State a point of view, or pattern?, What is the motive?		
Demonstrate, distinguish explain, give examples, match, paraphrase, show, summarize	students explain, state a rule, paraphrase, visual representation	Statement on words, What does it mean? , Give an example.. Explain what is happening, What is the main idea? Is this the same as...,? What are they saying? What seems likely?		
Choose, describe, find, identify, label, list, name, recall, recite, recognize	highlighting, memorizing, make a list, make a chart	Who?, Where?, What?, How?, When?, What does it mean?		

Figure 2.4 Revised Bloom's taxonomy

The second task is to use DOK to identify what the student has done as a result of the teacher question. In this example, the recorder would put a 1 in Quadrant 1.

The task is to see the relationship between the questions teachers ask (Revised Bloom's Taxonomy) and the student's outcome (DOK). The hope is for teachers to see that lower-level questions lead to lower-level student outcomes.

REFERENCES

Anderson, L. W. and Krathwohl, D. R., eds. (2001). *A Taxonomy for Learning, Teaching, and Assessing: A Revision of Bloom's Taxonomy of Educational Objectives*, complete edition. New York: Longman.

Bloom, B. S. (1956). *Taxonomy of educational objectives: The classification of educational goals, Handbook I: Cognitive Domain*. New York: David McKay.

Dewey, John. (1895). The Theory of Emotion. (1): Emotional Attitudes. *Psychological Review*, *1*, 553–569.

Dewey, John. (1896). The Reflex Arc Concept in Psychology. *Psychological Review*, *3*, 357–370.

Dewey, John. (1902). *The Child and the Curriculum*. Chicago: University of Chicago Press.

Dewey, John. (1902). *The School and Society*.

Dewey, John. (1916). The Relationship of Thought and Its Subject Matter, chapter 2 in *Essays in Experimental Logic*. Chicago: University of Chicago Press, pp. 75–102.

Dewey, John. (1933). *How We Think: A Restatement of the Relation of Reflective Thinking of the Educative Process*. Boston: D. C. Heath.

Dewey, John. (1938). *Experience and Education*. New York: Collier Books.

Ebbinghaus, Hermann. (1885). *Memory: A Contribution to Experimental Psychology* (Henry A. Ruger and Clara E. Bussenino, Trans.,1913). New York: Teachers College Press, Columbia University.

Hess, I. (2004). Applying Webb's Depth of Knowledge Levels in Reading. Online, available at www.nciea.org.

Holloway, John. (2000, November) How does the brain learn science? *Educational Leadership*, *58*(3): 85–86.

Hunter, M. (1979, October) Teaching is decision making. *Educational Leadership*.

Hunter, M. (1982). *Mastery Teaching*. El Segundo, CA: TIP Publications.

Webb, N. (1999). *Research Monograph No. 18: Alignment of Science and Mathematics Standards and Assessments in Four States*. Washington, D.C.: CCSSO.

Webb, N. (2005). Depth–of-Knowledge Levels for Four Content Areas. Presentation to the Florida Education Research Association, 50th Annual Meeting, Miami, Florida.

Webb, N. (1994, 2006). Research Monograph No. 6: Criteria for Alignment of Expectations and Assessments on Mathematics and Science education. Washington, D.C.: CCSSO.

Webb Alignment Tool (WAT) Training Manual, available at http://www.wcer.wise.edu/WAT/index.aspx.

Wolfe, Pat. (1999). Revisiting effective teaching. *Educational Leadership*, *56*(3), 61–64.

Wolfe, Patricia. (2001). *Brain Matters: Translating Research into Classroom Practice*. Alexandria, VA: Association for Supervision and Curriculum Development.

3

Using a Readiness Set

FOCUS OF THE CHAPTER

How to develop a Readiness Set to get the student's interest at the onset of a lesson or at the beginning of a new lesson. After the Readiness Set, the teacher plans the lesson to "make sense" and have meaning for the student. This phase is Stage 1 of the Pre-Delivery Stage: the Readiness Cycle.

INTRODUCTION

The Readiness Set has three components: the starter (or a catalyst, hook, attention getter), the connection of what will be taught to what students know; and the tie-in of the new information to the student's prior knowledge. Brain research promotes getting the student's attention and holding it, which is one purpose of a Readiness Set. The other purpose of a Readiness Set is to promote sense and meaning.

PROBING QUESTIONS

1. How will the teacher get her students interested in today's lesson?
2. How will the teacher focus student attention throughout the lesson?
3. What is forward and backward framing and how can it be used in instructional delivery?

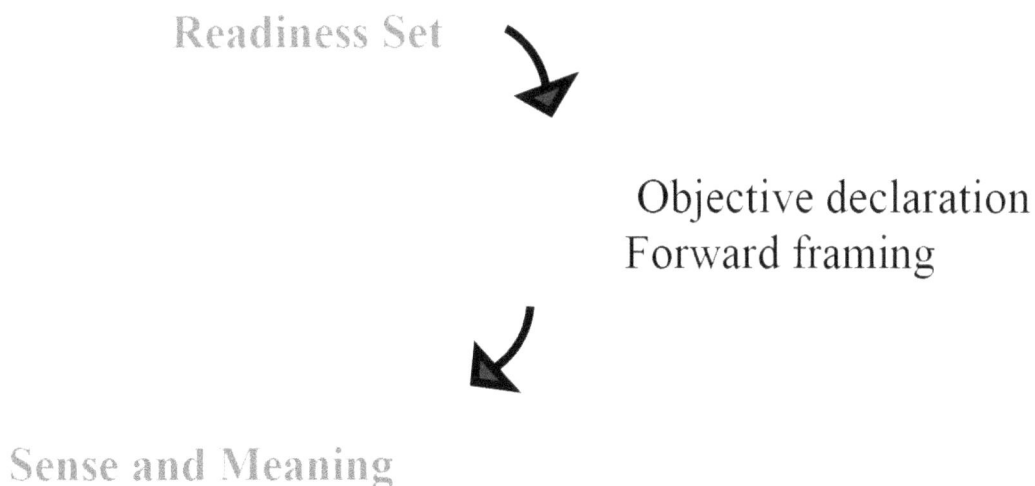

Readiness Set

Objective declaration
Forward framing

Sense and Meaning

Figure 3.1 Pre-delivery (readiness).

Table 3.1 Readiness Set Activity

Think of a lesson you will be teaching. Let's plan how to tie it to the student's frame of reference. First write the Student Learning Target (SLT) and Demonstration of Student Learning (DSL) for the lesson. SLT: DSL:
Starter: How will I start the Readiness Set? I must remember that the starter will ignite the student's interest, serving as an attention getter. The purpose is to set a "hook" into the student's interest. What interests my students? Since my students all have varied backgrounds, what do they have in common? Is there something in school that they all experience?
Connection: Once I have the student's interest, I have to show a connection to what will be taught. Remember the brain seeks patterns and connections, so making the connection for the student will facilitate the learning.
Tie-in: Connect the new knowledge with the student's frame of reference. Now that we have the student's interest and have made the connection, we tie it all together. For a person that fishes, it would be setting the hook and reeling in the prize, or completing the act.
After I use this Readiness Set, what would I change or keep the next time I use it?

Table 3.2 Using a Readiness Set Activity

Let's plan how to tie it to the student's frame of reference now that we have the Student Learning Target and Demonstration of Student Learning for the lesson.
Starter:
Connection:
Tie-in:
After I use this Readiness Set, what would I change or keep the next time I use it?

Reflection:

Readiness Set Group Activity

For this activity each teacher brings an objective and DSL to a meeting. They share their Readiness Set and ask for suggestions.

Table 3.3 Readiness Set Reflection Sheet

Subject _____ Grade level _____

Objective

DSL

Readiness Set

Subject _____ Grade level _____

Objective

DSL

Readiness Set suggestions:

The value of a Readiness Set is:

My best starters were:

because

My best connections were:

because

My best tie-ins were:

because

READINESS SET
BACKGROUND REFRESHER

Theorists such as John Dewey, Madeline Hunter, and Alfred North Whitehead focused their scientific learning theories and research on which teacher strategies positively affected and increased student learning in the classroom. In all cases, prior knowledge was important for student retention.

Pat Wolfe, founder of Mind Matters Inc., suggested that quite possibly the most effective teaching strategies of 20 years ago, such as Hunter and the earlier works of Dewey and Whitehead, are still relevant today because current cognitive and neuroscience research is continually proving the theories of the past to be instrumental in today's world of education.

Why Readiness Set

When new information is presented, our human brain immediately starts sifting and sorting through all of its sensory input, and simultaneously the brain searches through previously stored information, disseminating relevance of new information as potential hooks. A Readiness Set increases the possibility that the brain will search through the best networks and attend to the information that is meaningful for a particular topic or issue.

After the new information is presented, students need to practice and apply what they have learned. As the saying goes: How does one get to Carnegie Hall? Practice, practice, practice. Yes, practice is the answer but practice doesn't make perfect; one must do perfect practice to make perfect. Practice and repitition makes permanent.

The reason why practice makes permanent is that circuits or networks of neurons, when used repeatedly, get accustomed to firing together and eventually become hardwired and will fire automatically. This is an important concept for teachers to know when they give practice tasks to students. They must ensure that the work is done correctly so students do not reinforce incorrect information.

Research increases our understanding of why prior knowledge plays an important role in learning. It also helps us to better understand how and why the brain learns or doesn't learn. By gaining a scientific understanding of the brain, we can make better decisions about how to structure learning environments and instruction. With the integration of past learning theories and current brain research, educators can only maximize the potential of our students.

Education and the Readiness Set

At times, we have all heard a familiar tune and we think to ourselves, "I have heard that song before." The song may bring us back to a place and time that elicits fond memories. It may also bring us unhappy memories, but in any event, just remembering the time and place and its relationship to the tune is significant. We may have forgotten, over time, most of what we heard or felt, but once we return to that tune, the emotional memory pours back over us in an overwhelming state.

As teachers, we want to control the context in which information is presented. Most recently in education, there is even less control over content delivered to the students, due to the framework of many new teaching models. Teachers are willing to use the content in the best presentation possible, so that the objectives and principles of the lesson are clear and concise and so that students can retrieve the information and apply it when necessary. With regard to the constraints of educational framework, how is a teacher to promote information in a clear, concise way so that content becomes permanent?

Reflection Box: This makes sense because:

Readiness Activities

Activity 1: Readiness Set: What to Ask Yourself in Developing a Readiness Set

What Standards will be addressed?

How will the Student Learning Target address the standards?

How should I inform my students of the lesson's context and objective, in kid-friendly language?

What prior knowledge needs to be activated?

What do my students have in common that I can use for my Readiness Set?

What do the students need to know before they can delve into the lesson plan?

How will I know the lesson was successful?

Activity: 10 Readiness Sets

Here are 10 quick and effective strategies that are not only helpful, but easy to implement. As students become accustomed to the routine, you'll find that an effective Readiness Set will help your students launch into learning, on task and on time! Ask students to . . .

1. *Circle* the home-learning questions or problems they would like to discuss in class tomorrow. Have the students use the assignment as an entrance ticket to class. Once in class, the teacher selects students to read what they circled. Have a class discussion and during the discussion the teacher will get a better understanding of what the students know and need to know.

   Follow-up: Based on the discussion, give the students a list of key words to define from the passage that were problematic to most of the class and to come to class ready to discuss their findings. Students can add their own words to the list.

2. *Star* the homework questions or problems that are correct and explain why they are correct. Be prepared to begin class with your discussion. If there were any questions or concerns you had during the assignment, they will also be discussed in class.

   Follow-up: Have a chart of the most common starred words and ask students to explain why everyone felt they were key words

3. *Highlight* the main points in a previous lesson. Compare student highlights with main points the teacher has listed on the board. Have students use red, yellow, or green highlighter to identify unknown words, "not sure" words, or known words.

   Follow-up: Make a list of the red, yellow, and green words and use the red words as a

Readiness Set for the next day's lesson. **Or** *have students select red words they would like to research.*

4. *"In my own words."* Read a passage, *respond* briefly in writing to a passage, statement, or quotation. Be prepared to discuss your answer in class.

   Follow-up: Have the class take a pro and con position of what they read and come to class and talk to classmates who had pros and cons.

5. *Agree/Disagree.* When students come to class, ask them to list questions for which they agree/disagree. Ask students what the relationship is among the questions. The questions are all related to what the students would be studying for the daily lesson.

   Follow-up: After the agree/disagree list is presented, have students work in pairs (agree and disagree) to see if they can change the other person's vote. After the discussions, have a whole-group activity and share the correct answers to the questions. Students then research why the answers are correct.

6. *Detective.* Ask students to make a list of *key words* in the article they were given to read. Compare their list with the key words the teacher has listed on the board. Why is your list and the teacher list the same? Why is your list different from the teacher's list?

   Follow-up: Give the students a list of key words and ask them to play detective to determine why they were selected as key words.

7. *How does it apply?* After the teacher reads the Student Learning Target, she ask students to think about the practical application of the skill. Students are asked to quick-write two applications of the skill.

Follow-up: Tell the students that the DSL will be for them to explain their answer.

8. *T-Chart.* The teacher presents the Student Learning Target and on one side of the T-Chart students write what they know. The teacher presents information about the objective which students list on the other side to the T-Chart.

Follow-up: Students pair-share what they know and what they learned or teams can be formed.

9. *Graphic organizer.* Discuss the Student Learning Target with the class. Ask students to show what they know about the objective by using a graphic organizer. The teacher reviews the graphic organizers to get information about the student's frame of reference and prior knowledge. The teacher will use that information to develop a Readiness Set.

Follow up: The teacher provides a partially completed graphic organizer to the students and asks them to complete what they know and what they would like to know about the topic.

10. *Readiness Rose:* Using the graphic below as a visual for the students, the first picture is the Student Learning Target. The next picture represents the starter, sparkler, catalyst. The connection of student knowledge enhances the rose. How everything is tied together is the final picture.

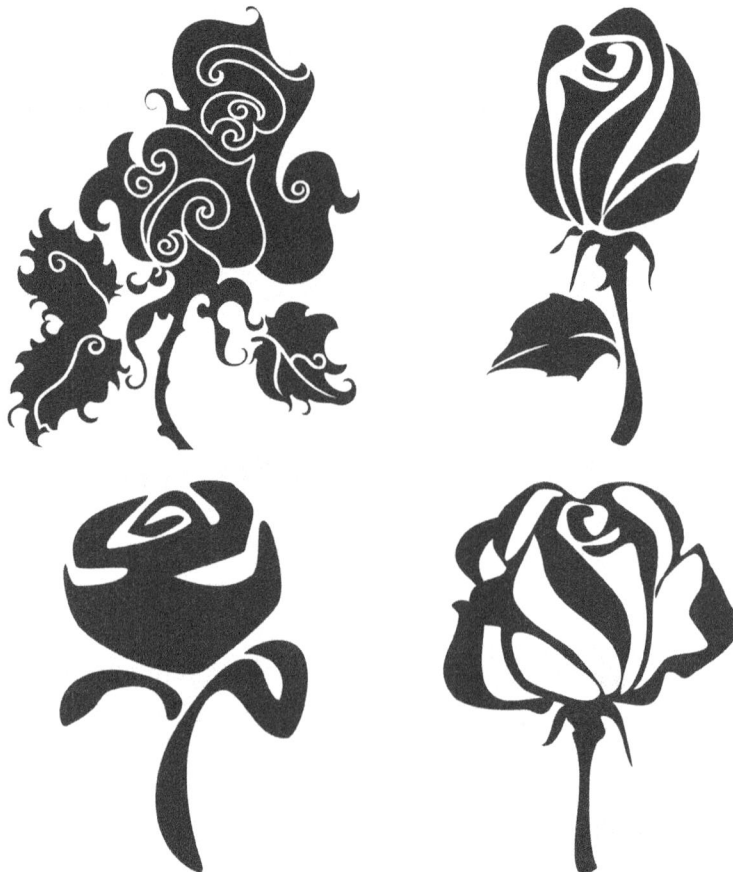

Figure 3.2 Roses https://www.istockphoto.com/vector/red-roses-sign-gm95361861-11297306.

This Workbook as a Readiness Set

Let's use this workbook as an example. The purpose of this workbook is to set the stage for what you wish to learn about the nature of the learner, instructional planning, and self-regulated learning. This workbook also gained your attention by eliciting a response from you based on your own experiences as both student and teacher. The introduction, pictures, and table of contents in this workbook hooked you into focusing upon what topics were to be presented in each chapter and, finally, it provided a framework for you to link prior knowledge to learning and make meaningful connections throughout your learning experience.

Readiness Set: Context Is Important

We remember information in the context in which it was presented. We may forget most of what we heard for a while, but once we hear the information again, it will prompt a memory for us. For example, we all have studied the Civil War and Abraham Lincoln. During the course of the study, we are presented information about Lincoln's assassination. That information was presented as an episodic incident, an incident that was presented and stored in our brains, until later when we retrieved it.

Ask someone if they remember the assassination of Dr. Martin Luther King Jr., or John F. Kennedy and most folks will remember studying about these two individuals, as there is meaning and significance attached to their names. Both Dr. King and JFK were connected to a movement or mindset and the information was not processed as an episodic event or a single event but in the context of a bigger frame of reference. As such, new information was attached to previous knowledge and the isolated information became more meaningful. It also helps to have an emotional attachment to the information as both Dr. King and JFK were loved by many people.

Combine the emotional attachment to the information and it becomes attached to memory.

Ways to Develop a Readiness Set

Teachers will engage students using a Readiness Set in two ways: one, using an auditory approach by providing an introduction—a "sparkler" or as a "catalyst" for what is to come so as to connect the student's prior knowledge; and, two, using a prop to add a visual component to the auditory approach.

Using a Prop Example

An effective way to focus the student and gain their interest is to use props. A prop is something used in creating or enhancing a desired effect. While students are reading the chapter book *The Cricket in Times Square* by George Selden (1960), a teacher might use a map of Grand Central Station, as a prop for a Readiness Set that introduces the setting of Times Square or a map of New York City that shows Times Square.

The prop will hook the student's interest and serve as a visual aid toward learning. The next step for the teacher is to isolate the prop in such a way so that a connection between the map of Grand Central Station / Times Square (or the map of New York City) and the chapter book depicting Times Square is made.

The teacher may state, "I have a picture on the whiteboard. Who can tell me about it?" The teacher waits for the responses from the students. Possible answers might be: "It's a map of Grand Central Station" or "It is a map of New York City showing Times Square." The teacher continues her questioning until the desired response is given.

Then the teacher states, "Correct. This is a picture of Grand Central Station." The teacher continues the questioning. "Has anyone ever been to Grand Central Station? What do you think happens there? Have you ever been to Times Square? Can you tell me what happens at Times Square? What happens at Times Square on New Year's Eve?" The teacher states, "It is a very popular station and it is near Times Square and that is where our chapter book story takes place."

The entire time the teacher is asking questions and soliciting answers from the students, she is keeping the visual aid prop on the whiteboard. At this point, the teacher will use the pen to circle the areas on the map that relate to the areas in the chapter book that are the same. The teacher continues her questioning as she works (or has a student identify the areas of NYC). She states, "Have you ever been to New York? Tell me what you liked about New York. Today we are going to read a story about Times Square."

When we read about a place that is familiar to you or that rings a bell in your head, raise your hand so that we can share your experience. Today's lesson is about making meaningful connections for you. When we do this together, we learn about each other and we can each gain understanding of our chapters in this fun-filled book!"

When the students read the chapter and raise their hand about the state of Connecticut or about a cricket, the teacher may use the whiteboard again to show that map. Or an innovative teacher may bring in a cricket box and the class could have a mascot while they are reading.

Many times local public libraries have interesting props that can be used for various pieces of literature. A prop can be homemade too. Anything that supports a lesson in some way is a prop. A word, a song, a movie clip, or even a one-liner joke, can be a support to a lesson that makes a connection for the student and uses another modality in presenting the information.

What If the Readiness Set Is Misused?

One way that a Readiness Set is misused is when it is called "review time." Unfortunately, in this case the Readiness Set is misunderstood and is not used properly to make the necessary connection to the lesson. The time that the Readiness Set is suppose to be presented is used to review homework, take attendance, pass out papers, or a variety of tasks not related to tying in prior knowledge. The notion of the Readiness Set is that it is not "review time" and instruction will begin after the review.

The point, however, is that the time used for a Readiness Set is specific and directed toward activating prior knowledge and not an opportunity to stimulate student interest with an unrelated task. The actual goal is to provide stimulus that relates in some way to the lesson content. Hook–Connect–Tie. Simply stated, hook the student's interest, connect the new information with the student's prior knowledge, and tie in everything with the lesson.

Reflection

MORE EXAMPLES OF READINESS SETS

A Readiness Set in a Kindergarten Lesson Plan

Topic: Patterns

Theme: There are patterns all around me. Can I identify them? Do I know what they are?

Objectives: I will be able to correctly identify four geometric shapes and three patterns in nature and everyday life.

Readiness Set: Teacher will use questions to probe student's prior knowledge and thereby gain an understanding of the student's background knowledge.

Teacher States:

"Who can name some things they saw on the way to school?" (*This ties in the student frame of reference.*) "What shapes were they?" (*This ties in the concepts of shapes to the outside world.*) "Look around the room and name some shapes that you see?" (*Teacher is focusing student attention to their surroundings outside school and their surroundings in the classroom. Teacher is also checking for learning by finding out what students made the connection to shapes that were discussed from the prior day's lesson.*) If children cannot name the shape on their own, ask them to "phone a friend" for the correct answer. Checking with students on shapes helps the students tie in their prior knowledge especially if the students actually see the shapes in the classroom or on the way to school.

Teacher States:

"Today we are going to continue our discussion about shapes in the classroom and then talk about shapes outside of the classroom."

Teacher prompts the students by questioning, "Yesterday we talked about different shapes which included: circle, square, triangle, rectangle, and octagon. Can someone give me examples of any one of the shapes you see in the classroom?" (*Teacher is stimulating prior knowledge.*)

"If I ask you what shape the clock is what would you say? What shape is the ceiling tile? What shape is the floor tile? What shape is the fire prevention sign? "What shape is the red stop sign by the door?" (*Examples of tying in student's prior knowledge from students with a variety of backgrounds or experiences.*)

Teacher States:

"Since we are identifying shapes in the classroom, let's think about the shapes outside the classroom. I know a few of you reported that you passed some houses on the way to school. Who said they passed Rahim's house? Great, let's close our eyes for a minute and visualize Rahim's house. If you didn't see Rahim's house, then visualize any house that you know about like your own" (*connections*).

I am going to get my pen and I am going to ask each one of you to come up to the whiteboard to draw all of the shapes that are in and on Rahim's house! Here we go!" The teacher continues to prompt the students with questions when they get "stuck." The teacher uses a drawing of Rahim's house as her on-going prop.

Examples: "What shape is his house?" (Students draw a square.) "Did it have a roof? What shape was the roof?" (Students draw a triangle.) "Now think hard about this one—how about the windows, what shape were they? Who would like to share something they saw and tell us what shape it is?"

Conclusion: The teacher checks for student understanding by evaluating the drawings on the whiteboard, as each child participates, and then asks the children to draw their own house on a piece of 8.5x11-inch paper and then evaluates the progress of each student. The teacher should remain consistent with the shape objective, but allow students to be creative. Within that creativity, it is hoped that the students will be noting that he or she is creating shapes as they draw.

Throughout the lesson, the teacher monitors student progress.

Note: The above questions and activities help to focus the student's attention (asking questions related to the classroom) and tie in the student's frame of reference (looking at shapes on the way to school or tying in a house of a classmates or their own) and tying it all together by reviewing shapes and then identifying them.

Additional Examples of Readiness Sets from A to Z

Analogy. Start the class with an analogy tied to the lesson. After the students see the analogy, have the students make their own analogy. Discuss student analogies.

A is to B   C is to X

Ask a Question; Get an Answer. Pose a question to the class and have students write an answer to the question posed. Use the question as readiness for the lesson. Alternative: send a question, get an answer.

Q & A form

Q

A

Brainstorm. Have students share their contextual knowledge about the Student Learning Target.

The sharing will allow the students to tap into their prior knowledge before teaching the new concept.

A & Q form

A

Q

Bubble Map

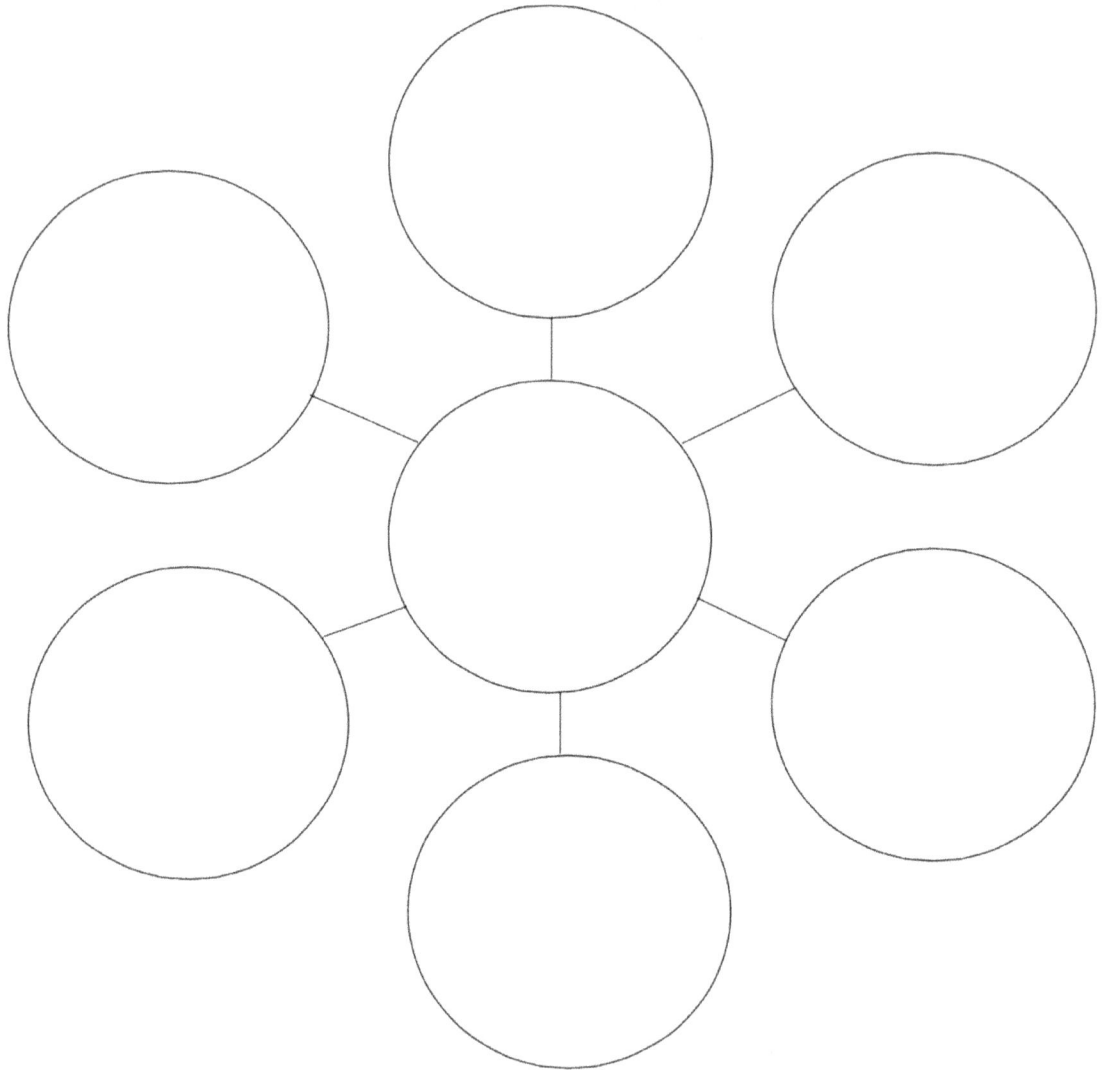

Figure 3.4 Bubble map.

Funnel. After the Student Learning Target is posed, have students add what they know. The added comments will be discussion points until one final solution is determined.

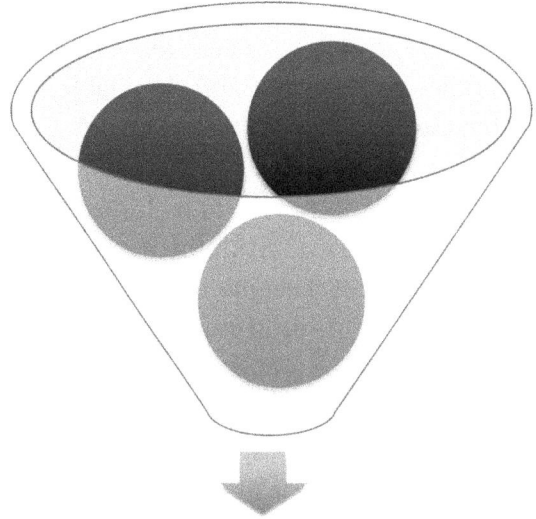

Figure 3.5 Funnel.

Challenge. Present a challenge question to the class. The challenge question is actually readiness for the lesson. Ask the class to deduce how two items are related. After a discussion, provide an example tied to the new lesson.

Close the Loop. After the Readiness Set is introduced and the lesson is taught, students do a reflection sheet on what they learned and if it all made "sense" to them and had meaning. The students show their "closed loop" the next day for teacher review.

Experiment. Conduct an experiment that illustrates a concept. For example, use water to fill 3D containers to illustrate volume or help students make a recipe using benchmark measurements. Have students write the process used to solve the problem.

Gallery Walk. Teacher places a note pad in each corner of the room, posting a different question related to what the students will be studying. Divide class into four groups. Each group will spend a few minutes at each station, read the comments, and add their comments. The original group will report on the comments made by the other groups and lead a discussion. The goal is for students to come to a conclusion related to a particular concept.

Graphic Organizer. Provide students with a graphic organizer based on thoughts closely related to the learning objective. For factual information the students can use a T-Chart; to compare and contrast, they can use a Venn diagram; to show understanding they can use thought clouds. After they complete the chart, students can pair-share their information. The teacher can use the information to assess student learning or readiness for the lesson.

How Does This Apply? Use a prop from a story students are about to read and have them tell you how it applies.

I Have a Challenge/Riddle. Prior to introducing a new concept, give students a challenge or problem to solve. Using inquiry can engage students and motivate them to learn.

Make a Prediction. Prior to teaching a lesson, have students make a prediction based on a few facts that the teacher presents.

Manipulatives or Models. Use physical models to prepare students to learn a specific concept or better highlight the critical attributes of new concepts. The model will serve as talking points for the lesson.

News Reporter. Present information to the class and ask them to write a news release based on the information. Have resources available for the students to use.

Prop. Use a prop to tweak student interest in the material to be covered. Ask probing questions to the students so they become interested in seeing the relationship of the prop to what they are seeing and what they will be studying.

Play a Game. Playing a quick game in order to recall prior knowledge can be an effective strategy for getting students engaged in the lesson and prepared to build off prior knowledge.

An example: Play a quick math-facts game, such as "around the world" prior to introducing multi-digit multiplication.

Pro/Con/Not Sure. Pose questions to the class about the topic to be taught. After the students cast their vote of agree, disagree, or not sure, have them discuss their reasoning in their groups. After the discussion have student try to convince folks who do not agree with them to come to their team. After a discussion, the teacher provides factual information to the questions posed.

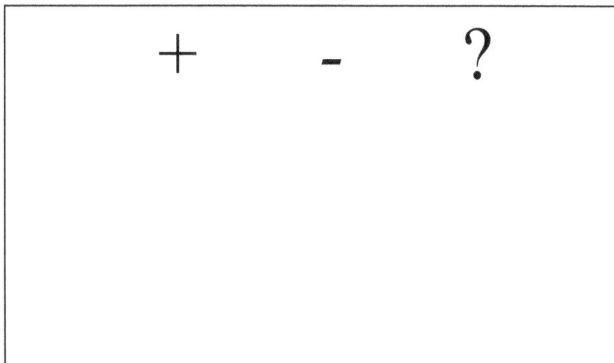

Readiness Set Story Walk. Tell your class that they are going on a Story Walk. Prior to reading a story, show the students the text and ask them to make predictions about the plot, the characters, and the story itself. After reading the story, have the students identify supporting details and assess whether their predictions were correct. A great introduction to the lesson is making predictions. After a short period of time, pull the class together and have them discuss their findings. Ensure that although they made predictions, their facts are correct.

Song or Video Clip. There are a wide variety of songs and video clips available for use in the classroom to prime the students' interest on the subject. Using songs and clips can be a way of drawing in students to show the relationship of music to culture.

Story. Tell a story directly to the material. Remember stories are psychologically privileged, that is, the brain will remember stories. If a story is told, make sure it is related to what you want the students to remember.

Survey. Survey your students by asking questions and having them step to a side or corner of the room that represents their response. After a brief discussion, have the students develop their own survey questions to ask the class.

Tweet. Have students tweet information about their home-learning assignment. Review the tweets and decide which are factual and which need more data. Provide direct instruction based on the tweets to enhance students' frame of reference.

Venn Diagram from their analogy. As the lesson progresses, have the students track similarities and differences of the new skills with prior skills.

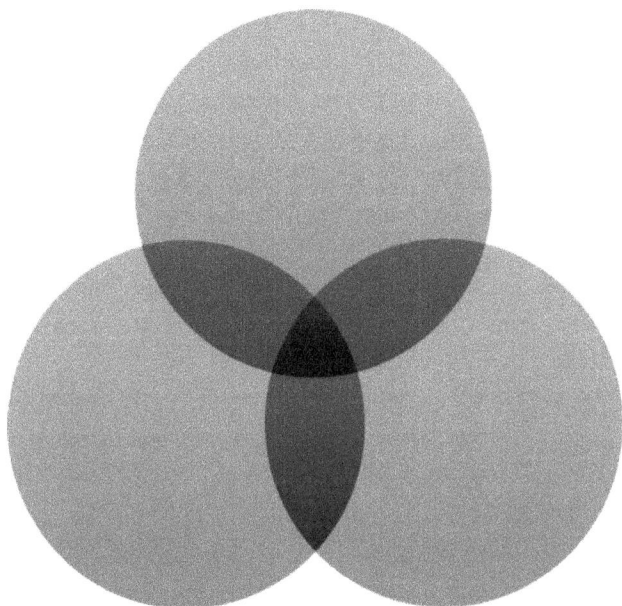

Figure 3.3 Venn diagram.

What's the Connection? Give students a group of words related to the lesson. Have them guess the topic or find the word that doesn't fit in the group. Students write the connections among the words. *What's the Connection? Tell a Story.* The teacher lists words on the whiteboard. Students write the connection between the words that the teacher listed. The students then write a story based on the words and connection.

Writing Prompt. Ask students to write everything they know about the posted Student Learning Objective, or present them with a prompt that is closely related to the Student Learning Objective.

BRAIN RESEARCH RELEVANT TO THE READINESS SET

Summary

1. Review of previous material to stimulate prior knowledge is critical for long-term learning.

2. Ask questions to stimulate student predictions as questions promote student metacognition. When students make predictions, dopamine is released when they are correct. The dopamine rush causes a pleasurable feeling and a pleasurable feeling makes a connection for the child.

3. A safe student environment is conducive to a positive school climate. A safe school environment is also necessary for students to feel comfortable to guess or to try new activities.

4. Ask students questions related to their personal experiences or frame of reference (their classroom, their home, a friend's home) to help them see relationships.

5. Tying the new lesson to their school experience ensures that all students will have a frame of reference tied to school. Students may have different home experiences, but they all come to school and have common experiences in the school or their classroom.

6. The Readiness Set creates patterns, contexts, and relevance to help the student's brain understand connections.

7. The use of a prop to gain attention only makes the brain connection stronger in the Readiness Set.

8. The Readiness Set begins the process of activation of student prior knowledge.

9. The Readiness Set begins the process of self-regulation.

REFERENCES

Dewey, John. (1897). *My Pedagogic Creed*, available online at http://www.rjgeib.com/biography/credo/dewey.html

Dewey, John. (1897). The psychology of effort. *Philosophical Review, 6.*

Dewey, John. (1910). *How We Think.* Lexington, MA: D. C. Heath.

Dewey, John. (1913). *Interest and Effort in Education.* Riverside Educational Monographs. Boston: Houghton Mifflin.

Dewey, John. (1930, July 9). How much freedom in new schools? New *Republic, 63*.

Dewey, John. (1933). *How We Think: A Restatement of the Relation of Reflective Thinking to the Educative Process*. Boston: D. C. Heath.

Dewey, John. (1938). *Experience and Education*. New York: Collier Books.

Hunter, M. (1982). *Mastery Teaching*. El Segundo, CA: TIP Publications.

Hunter, R., and Hunter, M. C. (2004). *Madeline Hunter's Mastery Teaching: Increasing Instructional Effecti vess in Elementary and Secondary Schools*. Thousand Oaks, CA: Corwin Press.

Kaufman, E. F., Robinson, J. S., Bellah, K. A., Aviers, C. A., Haase-Wittler, P., and Martindale, L. (2008). Engaging students with brain-based learning. *Techniques: Connecting Education & Careers, 83*(6).

Kitchel, T., and Tones, R. M. (2005). Meaning as a factor of increasing retention. Proceedings of American Association for Agricultural Education, National AAAE Research Conference, May 25–27, San Antonio, Texas,

Pollock, Jane E. (2007). *Improving Student Learning One Teacher at a Time*. Alexandria, VA: Association for Supervision and Curriculum Development.

Whitehead, Alfred North. (1978). *Process and Reality*. New York: The Free Press.

Whitehead, Alfred North. (1929). *The Aims of Education and Other Essays*. New York: Macmillan.

Wolfe, Pat. (1999). Revisiting Effective Teaching. *Educational Leadership, 56*(3), 61–64.

Wolfe, Patricia. (2001). *Brain Matters: Translating Research into Classroom Practice*. Alexandria, VA: Association for Supervision and Curriculum Development.

4

Developing Sense and Meaning

FOCUS OF THE CHAPTER

Developing sense and making meaning are required if information is to be stored into long-term memory. Sense and meaning are part of the "Readiness Stage "of the Learner's Brain Model. This chapter addresses how to use cues, prompts, reinforcement, and note taking to promote making sense and developing meaning for the student. Activities will be provided.

INTRODUCTION

How is making "sense" and promoting "meaning" developed? Why is sense and meaning necessary in the informational stage and for the closing stage? How is sense and meaning developed at each phase of this stage? The various phases in the sense and meaning process will be discussed in the chapter.

PROBING QUESTIONS

1. What is the role of making sense and having meaning for a lesson?
2. How can I use cues, prompts, and gestures to focus student attention throughout the lesson?
3. What are student "killer questions"?
4. How will I promote reflection to use for student self-regulation?

Bridging new and prior information

Cues

Prompts

Transfer

Reinforcement

Reflection

Note taking

Figure 4.1 Sense and meaning.

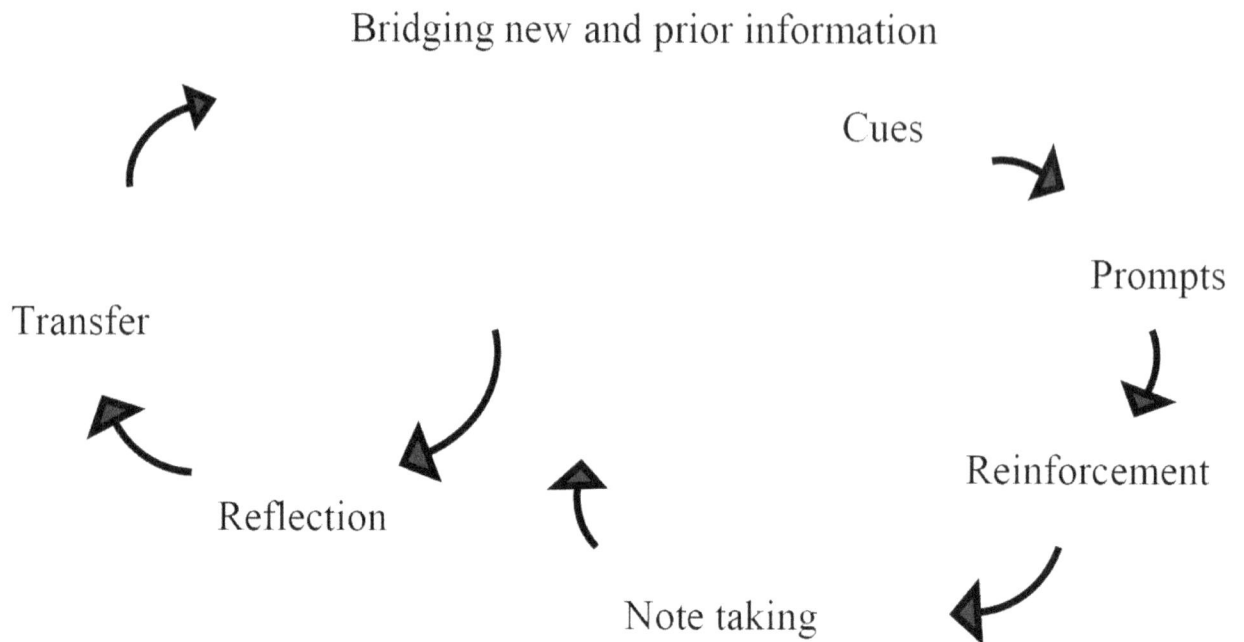

Does the figure make sense?

Why not?

What would you add?

Activity for Sense and Meaning: What Are Student "Killer Questions"?

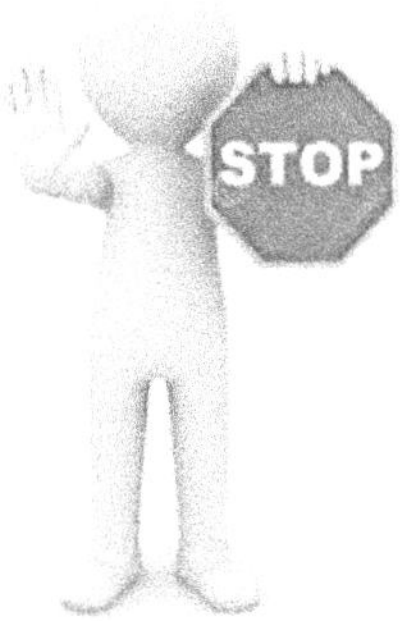

What do I do when students ask "killer questions"

_____

_____

_____

_____

_____

_____

_____

_____

_____

_____

_____

Figure 4.2 Activity for sense and meaning.

Sense and Meaning

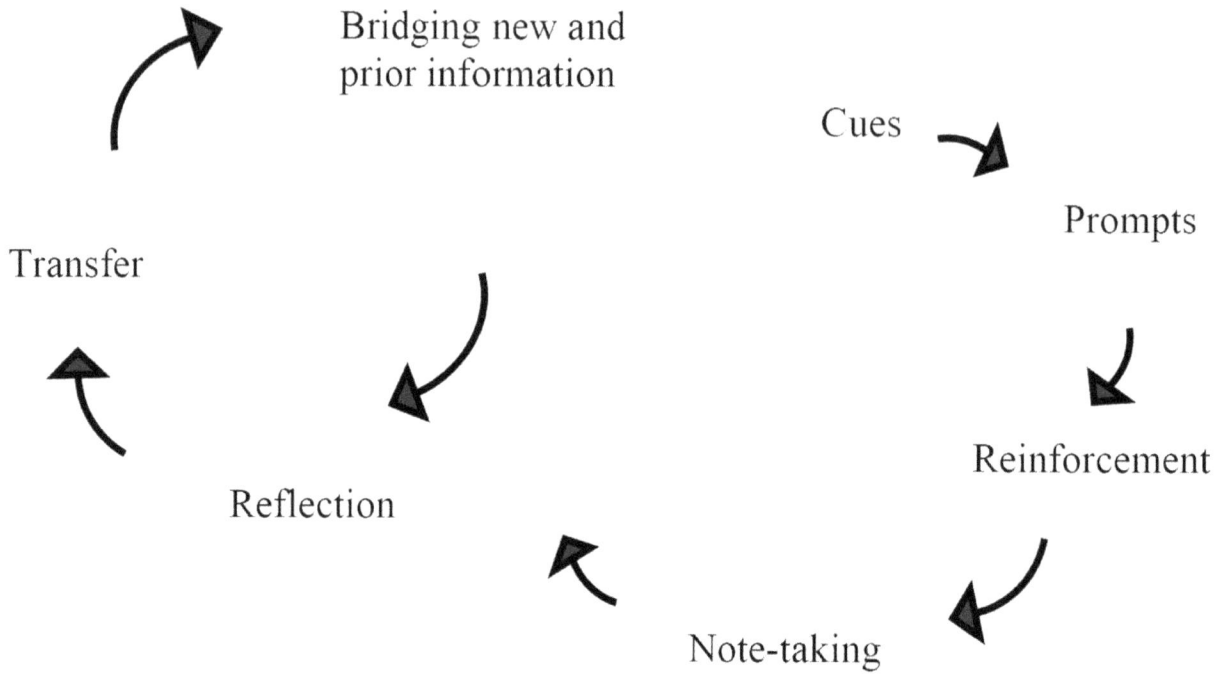

Bridging new and
prior information

Cues

Prompts

Transfer

Reinforcement

Reflection

Note-taking

Figure 4.3 Sense and meaning.

How do I use cues, prompts and gestures to focus student attention throughout the lesson?

What is my favorite focusing question?

RESEARCH ON SENSE AND MEANING

The Sense and Meaning Question: Tell Me Why We Are Studying This?

Why are we studying this? Will we be able to use this information? Will this be on the test? These are some of the many questions teachers are asked by students while teachers are presenting lessons. These types of questions send a powerful message to the teacher, which translates into the fact that the student does not see the value or the usefulness of the lesson's subject matter and that what is being taught does not make sense to the student. Additionally, this tells the teacher that the information presented has little or no meaning to the student.

The human brain searches for sense and meaning. Teachers need to offer a variety of approaches and resources to allow for students to make sense and develop meaning, see patterns for developing relationships, and transfer the new knowledge into real-world application. In essence, the utility of what they are learning.

How does the teacher facilitate the learning so that the student understands the relationship of the subject matter to his or her own frame of reference? In addition, how will the teacher facilitate the desired outcome, so that this outcome results in students making meaning and a positive connection to the brain of the student?

SENSE AND MEANING ACTIVITIES

One way to help students connect with their learning or to develop sense and meaning is to use an activity known as the "What and How." The "What and How" is a useful classroom assessment tool for prompting student application of learned material. The process begins when the teacher identifies a principle, theory, or generalization for the student or when the student has read about an important principle, theory, or procedure in class. The objective is to focus on what is being learned and prompt the students to connect new ideas to prior knowledge, think creatively, and use the connections. "The What" is the material learned and "The How" is its application. A t-chart can be used for this activity.

Table 4.1 What and How Activity

"What" — What are the critical attributes, principles, or main concepts of the material?	"How" — How can the main points be applied?
What Example: Today's skills are: In geometry we are learning about area. We will learn about measuring, recording the data, drawing a proposed garden, and calculating area.	How application: My Uncle Guido wants me to plan a garden with tomato plants. The land is in the shape of a rectangle and the plants have to be 75cm apart. Using the skills we learned today, compute how many plants can be planted in the garden.
"What"	"How"

Reflection

To help students see relationships and make meaning they do a "Bubbles" activity.

Write a main concept or principle above the bubbles, which is the center of the Bubble. How is the principle connected to the other bubbles?

Main Principle

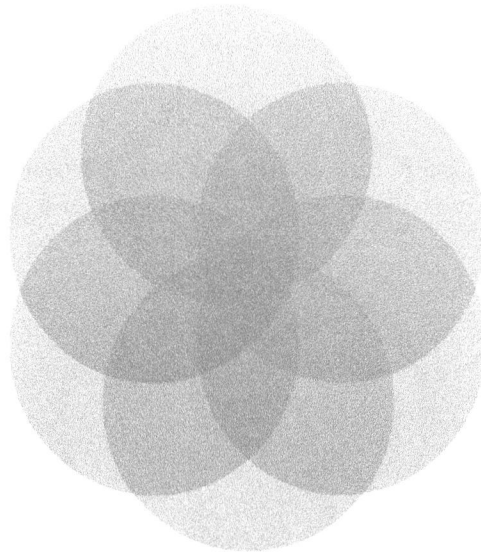

Figure 4.4 Bubbles activity.

Reflection

Students use a graphic organizer to show connections or how everything makes "sense."

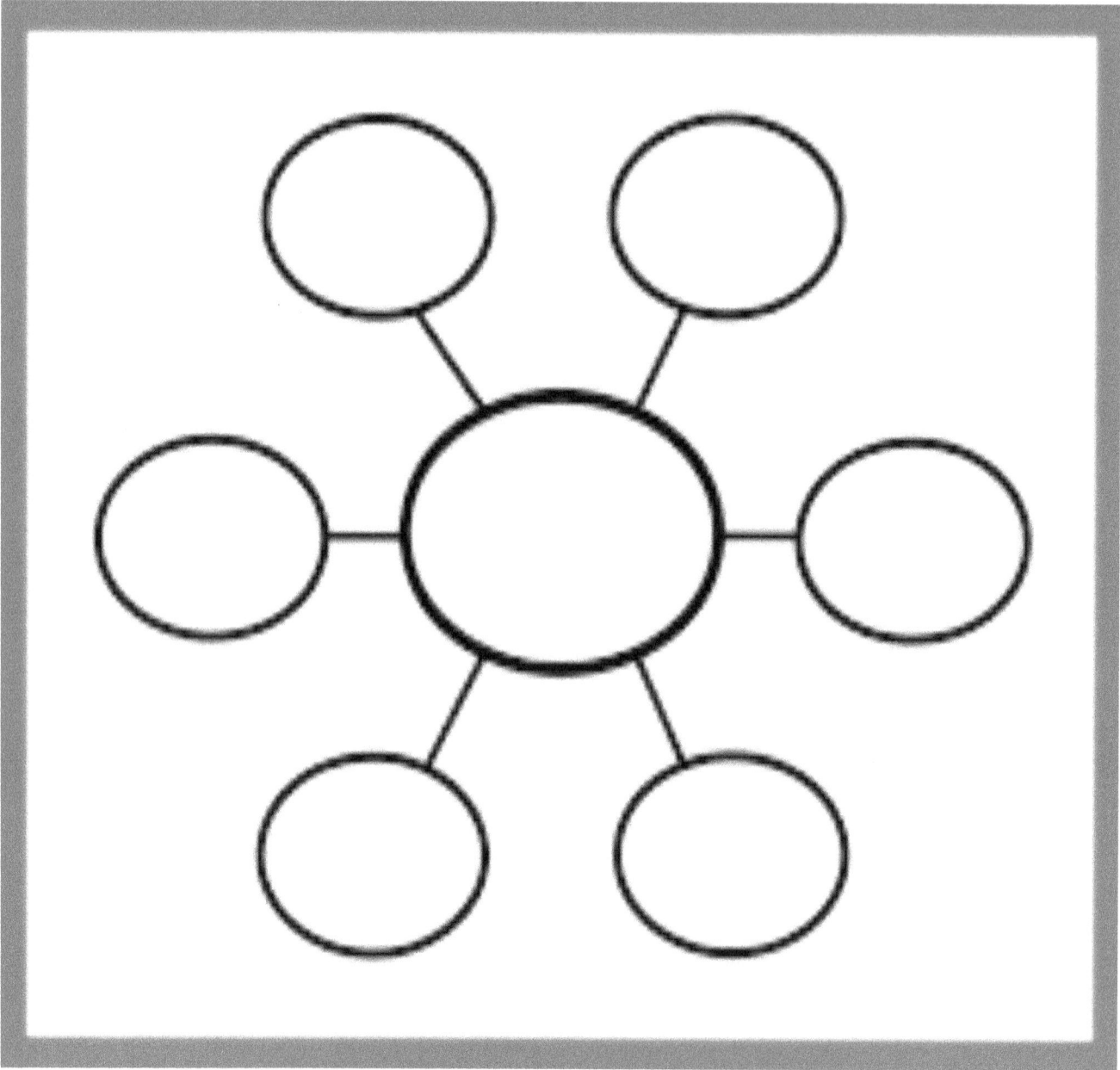

Figure 4.5 Graphic organizer.

Reflections: What Do I Notice?

Students use a rosebud to describe why everything makes sense because of the interrelationships.

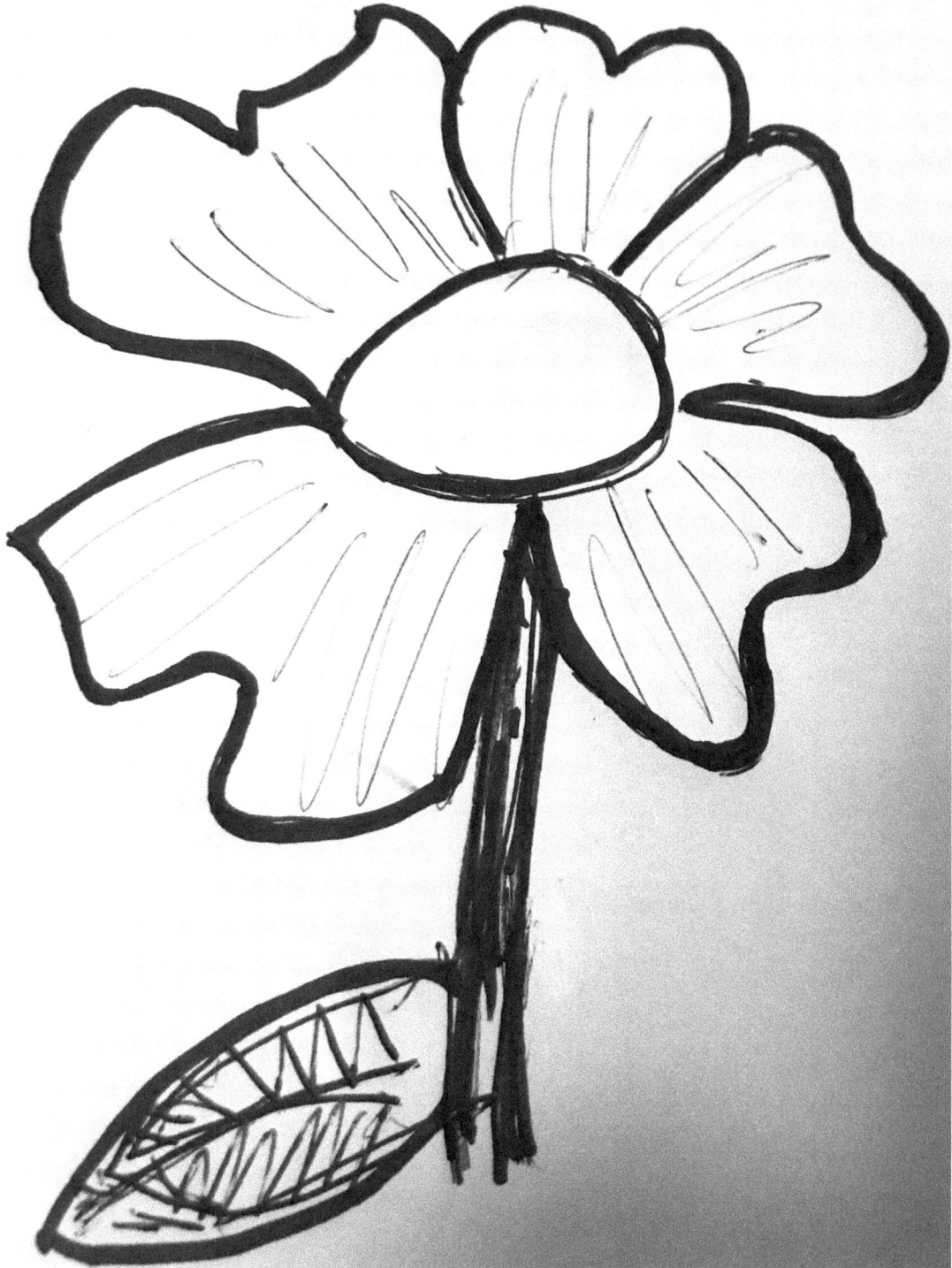

Figure 4.6 Rosebud.

Reflections: What Do I Notice?

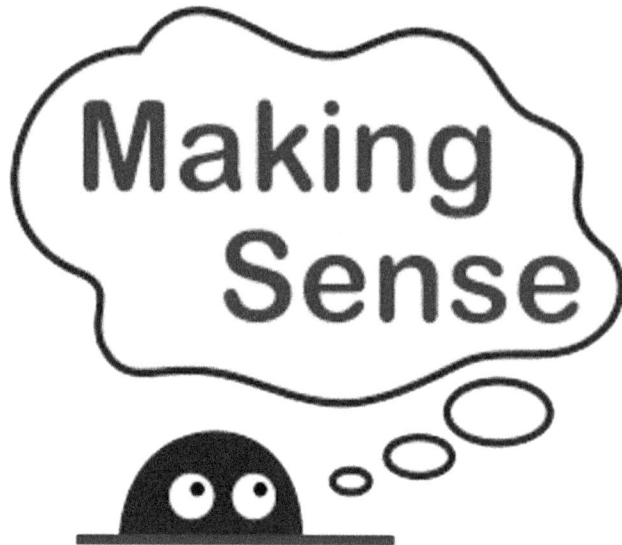

Figure 4.7 Making sense.

The lesson makes sense because:

I will be able to use the skills I learned

Instructional Strategies to Promote Deeper Meaning

Meaning List is a strategy whereby the teacher will list words on the whiteboard that describe what will be learned. The teacher references these descriptions throughout the lesson, so that the students will be able to connect the key points being discussed to the Student Learning Target. To be effective, the teacher must refer back to the key words and/or ask students to discuss among their peers what the key words mean to them.

Alternative: Throughout the lesson, the students develop a "meaning list" of words they feel are important. The put their list on a 3 x 5 index card and use it as an exit ticket from the class.

What I know. The assessment directs the teacher to prepare three open-ended or multiple-choice questions. Students are then instructed to answer the questions that are posed to them. Based on the information received from the students, teachers can proceed with the lesson. In addition, throughout the lesson the teacher can refer back to questions that he or she posed to the student.

The teacher may ask, "What are we learning today? Remember the key points that we will be discussing today; how do they apply to the real world?" To promote further student engagement, students should work in pairs to determine meaning, usefulness, and application throughout the lesson. This pair-share model encourages brainstorming and connections which will lead to better learning and application. These questions posed by the teacher can also be used as a "hook" to engage the students and spark an interest in the subject matter.

Exit Ticket: My Meaning List

Student name _____

Class period _____

My "meaning" list of words from today's lesson are:

Words:

Reason why I think they are important:

Teacher feedback:

Exit Ticket: What I Learned

Student name _____

Class period _____

Student Learning Target:

What I know:

What I learned:

Teacher feedback:

Realignment is when one applies the correct stem to an appropriate question. For example, a student states one application of Newton's third law (for every action there is always an opposite and equal reaction) and then gives an example of how it is applicable in the real world.

The onset of the process begins when the teacher first indicates that the law, which was stated, was Newton's second law and not the third law. The student then sees the teacher's correction and is able to correctly attach the application answer to the correct principle. Realignment is necessary otherwise the student will not understand the appropriate relationship between the stem and the answer. It helps to make sense and develop appropriate meaning.

Why is a method by which the learner questions or internalizes the presented material. The process of the interrogation involves asking students to think beyond facts by questioning each fact with a why statement to construct reasons why the factual relationships make sense.

By the third "why" students are getting deeper and deeper into developing understanding. Peter Senge (2006) uses five whys as a method to dig deep but experience has taught me that my frustration level at the fifth why was pretty high, consequently using three whys for students may be more reasonable. If not, the teacher can move from three whys to five whys.

Connection List is another method, in which the teacher will list words on the whiteboard that describe what will be learned or, in other words, details the objective of the lesson. The teacher references these descriptions throughout the lesson, so that the students will be able to connect the key points being discussed to the new learning objective. To be effective, the teacher refers back to the "connection" words and/or asks students to discuss among themselves how the key words are connected. Students write a three-sentence summary of how the words are connected.

Exit Ticket:
The Why Game

Student name _____

Class period _____

Today the teacher taught [Student Learning Target]: It is important because:

Why

Why

Why

Exit Ticket:
Connections List

Teacher words [Teacher lists key words that will be discussed in the lesson.]	Answers [Teacher provides possible answers but lists more answers than words so students will have options and not rely on the process of elimination.]

SCHEMA FOR SENSE AND MEANING

Developing sense and meaning is the beginning of the "Readiness Phase" in the Learner's Brain Model. In this phase, the student will be acquiring knowledge to be used at a later time. Stages for helping students to remember are: recording (acquisition of information); retaining (storage—short- or long-term storage); and retrieving (retrieval of the information upon demand).

To help remember these phases think of a file cabinet. In the first stage, one acquires the information. One acquires "files" or bits of information. After information is acquired (acquisition stage) it is retained or filed (storage stage) in the file cabinet, under the appropriate category. Finally, when information is secured and requested, the file is retrieved from the file cabinet.

Use the space below to draw *My Model of Sense and Meaning*.

Sense and Meaning

Bridging new and
prior information

Use of Cues to promote cognition

Practice and application

Prompt reinforcement

Cognitive

Connection

Transfer of meaning via sense making
and application

Reinforcement or realignment

Transfer of knowledge via making meaning

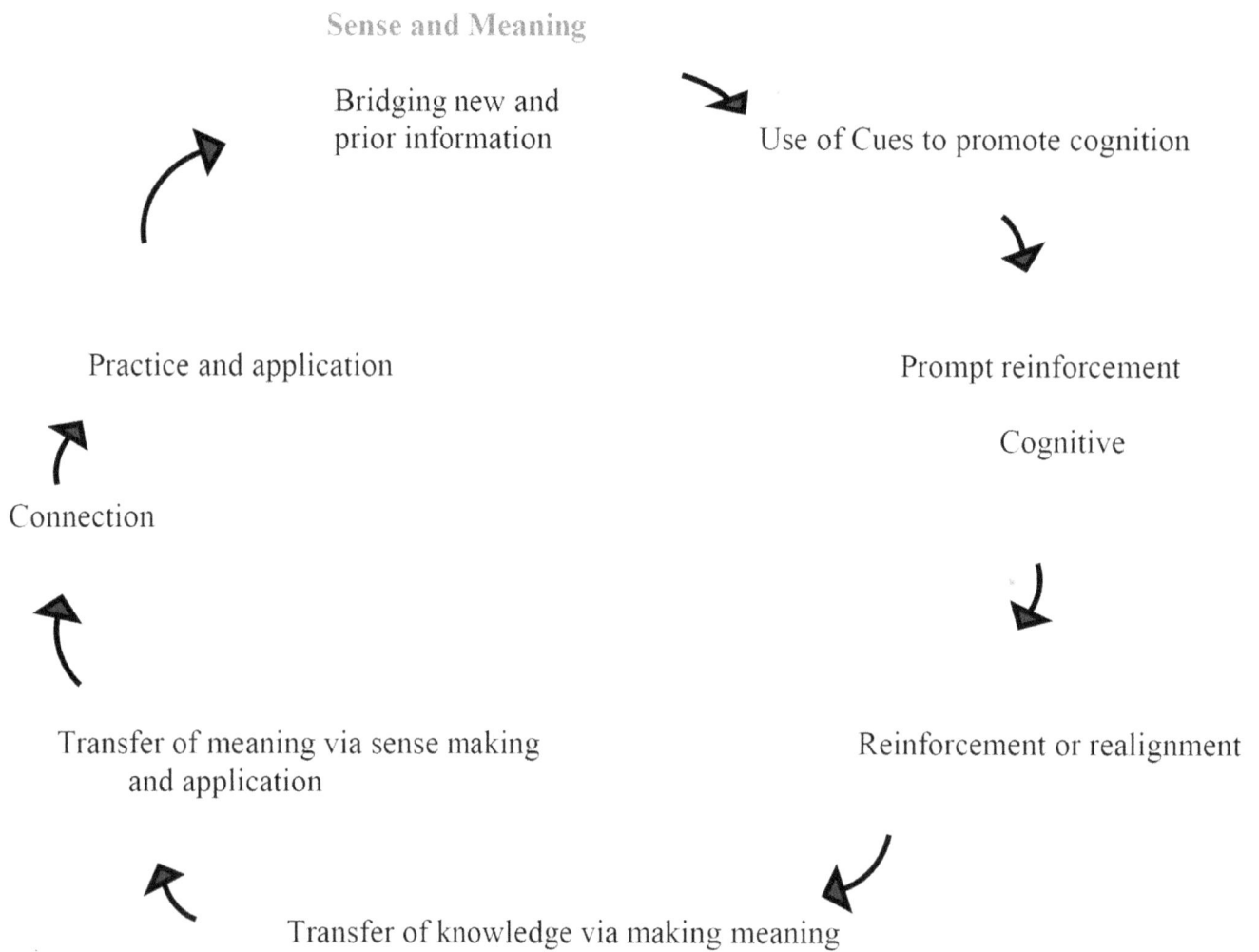

Figure 4.8 Schema for sense and meaning.

Transfer of Knowledge via Making Meaning

Is each phase needed for the schema? If so, why? If not, why not?

Is Your Model of Sense and Meaning the same or different that the Schema for sense and meaning in Figure 4.8?

Sense and Meaning as It Relates to the Readiness Stage

Readiness, the first stage of instructional delivery, is defined as the preparation of the students toward learning. In order to prepare a student, it is necessary to activate the student's prior knowledge, so that the material being presented will have relevance and meaning to the student.

Ways to Promote Sense and Meaning in the Readiness Stage

Using gestures, visual and auditory prompts, praise, and cues during class instruction to scaffold children's learning in the spirit of guided participation are ways teachers have to guide student thinking and understanding. It is also a way to ensure student participation.

Prompting

This prompting process helps to focus attention and to develop meaning. By a scaffolding question, the teacher prompts the student to begin the process of metacognition. For instance, "Have you considered . . . ?" The teacher develops higher-level questions, so the student can analyze, interpret, synthesize, and form new conclusions. The questioner should develop analytical questions that illicit inferences, analyze supporting or conflicting information, and develop a personal perspective, based on his or her reasoning. Lower-level questions can be used to bring the student to a higher level.

Depending on how the student answers, the teacher may continue prompting the students and encourage them to dig deeper into the work. Often students will have a chart to collect stickers and rewards as a visual aid and external positive reinforcement. The verbal praise should be an observation of what the student is doing and how well that student is doing the task. External and internal reinforcement is important.

Giving Feedback to Students

Based on the feedback the student receives, the teacher will reevaluate her method of instruction and decide what changes need to take place such as continue the lesson, re-teach the skill, or end the instruction and start all over. The feedback given by the teacher will help the student frame the information received and determine its value.

Assuming teachers understand that a climate of trust in the classroom is important, the teacher ensures the development of the climate of trust and mutual respect. The goal is to create an atmosphere for students that promotes engagement. One way this can be done is for the teacher to engage students in dialogue and make them feel that their opinions are respected. Another way to develop a trust relationship is for the teacher to understand the value of feedback and how feedback is provided to the student.

Important considerations for providing feedback are:

1. Feedback should be corrective in nature. The goal is to provide guidance for reflection and improvement.
2. Feedback should be timely. Feedback loses its effect if it is delayed or given at a later time or date.
3. Feedback should be specific.
4. Feedback can be peer generated, but if it is, it must be based on standards or a rubric or it becomes an opinion.
5. Students can effectively provide their own feedback as part of a self-regulation process. Teachers can evaluate the feedback to see if the students are "on track."

The teacher's comment must be clearly paired to the desired behavior or the specific action. To acknowledge a positive situation the teacher must first observe a specific behavior (i.e., the student is reading a chapter book quietly without disturbing others) and then tell the student exactly what he or she is doing correctly. Once the teacher has noted the specific observable behavior, then she can add positive recognition to the behavior. For example, the teacher may state, "X, I see that you are reading your chapter book. You certainly are focused and your neighbors must think what a great role model you are for them."

This kind of comment will demonstrate to the student immediate clarity, recognition for positive behavior, and set up chapter book expectations for the future. By using this positive reinforcement strategy, the teacher will maintain classroom management with ease. Building a classroom of positive feedback in this fashion will begin to extinguish negative behaviors.

I have discussed many different strategies to focus the student in this chapter. There are many more stated and described in detail in the book *Setting the Stage: Teaching to the Learner's Brain Using the Learner's Brain Model*. The next important topic I wish to discuss that is useful is note taking.

Exit Ticket: The Why Game (Tell Grandma)

Student name _____

Class period _____

Today the teacher taught [Student Learning Target]: It is important because:

Why

Why

Why

Tell Grandma card

NOTE TAKING

If note taking is an important strategy for learning, then what are the principle functions of it? What strategies are employed? How can note taking be used to facilitate learning? And more importantly, how can note taking be taught as an essential skill?

The primary function of note taking is to record what is being presented, so that the notes can assist at a later date for study skills. Writing verbatim—exactly what is being said—is the least effective way to take notes. Note taking is a process that the student must learn. If students record every word that the teacher is saying, it will not allow them to synthesize information into the brain and will not enable them to make sense or develop meaning about what was discussed during the lesson.

To help promote note-taking skills, one system for students to employ is Cornell's Note Taking Method. This technique is very useful for the student, as it allows her to use the notes to study and reflect upon what was taught. There is also a note-taking review sheet which can be used to help the student make sense and develop meaning from the notes.

Remember note taking is more that just a process for the student to use. The notes are to be used as review and study material so the student must review the notes to see if what she wrote made sense or needs to be refined. The real value is taking the notes and seeing how the information can be applied. If the information can not be applied, then note taking was an exercise in writing and not skill building.

Reaction:

Table 4.4 Note Review Handoug

Note Summary: Summarize your notes in three sentences or in a bulleted list of words
Reflection: The notes make sense because:
Reflection: The notes have meaning because:
I can apply the notes when I:
Overall reflection

Value of Note Taking

Note taking is important as students can use their notes to study and better understand the value of the material they learned. Note taking enhances lecture learning by activating attention mechanisms and engaging the learner's cognitive processes of coding, integrating, synthesizing, and transforming orally received input into a personal and meaningful form.

Note taking is beneficial because the recorded notes serve as an external repository of information that permits later revision and review. The review process helps to stimulate the recall of information.

Generalizations Regarding Note Taking

The least effective way to take notes is verbatim. Attempting to record everything that is heard or read does not give students a chance to synthesize the information presented. This does not suggest that students should take limited notes; in fact, the more notes the students take, the better. It is important, however, that notes be specific to the learning goals outlined by the teacher.

Students should consider notes as "dynamic" or a work in progress. They are a work in progress because they should be reviewed, revised, and amended to take into account additional information received from the teacher or gathered by the student.

Students should use the notes as study guides, highlighting specific words or concepts to form a structural understanding of the material.

Ensure that notes are clear, well-organized, and easy to read.

Notes should be used for review and study not just an activity to put in a trapper or binder.

Teacher Strategies to Support Note Taking

One strategy is pacing. Pacing is an important tool that enables the teacher to help the student process information. If there is a lot of technical information and/or terminology in the lesson, the teacher should be mindful of how fast or slow she is delivering the information to allow ample time for the student to process what is being presented. The teacher should use frequent checks for understanding to ensure that the students know the terminology.

Set the pace and flow of the information being presented in accordance with the student's readiness and ability. If the student has a strong foundation of knowledge and comprehends the facts, then the teacher should do checks of understanding, or spot evaluations to determine if she can possibly hasten the pace of the lesson or if she should slow the pace of the lesson.

Another way to adjust the pace during note taking is to pause during the lesson. A pause, or hiatus, during the lesson helps slow down the pace of the delivery. The teacher can build in "break points" during the lesson, and ask the students to explain what they just learned. To be better prepared, the teacher can build the questions she intends to ask. The questioning process will set the stage for helping the students make connections in the subject matter so the brain sees a pattern.

There are also several strategies that can be used to slow the pace of the lesson, which aids note taking. The teacher can ask the students to pick keywords from the discussion and then share their keywords with the rest of the class. These keywords are heard and remembered by the students.

It is also very important for the teacher to record the key words visually on a chart as the students recite, out loud in class, key words that they found. By listening, speaking, and writing the keywords, the teacher is differentiating lesson delivery using a variety of learning preferences for all of her students, resulting in focused attention and memorization.

Another way to pace the lesson is to provide a list of words to the students. While the teacher is instructing the lesson, she will be using the keywords.

When one of the words is heard within the lecture, the students will be asked to define the word. The class will then engage in a discussion about the definition the classmate proposed. After the class discussion, students will develop a whole "class" definition. This process will slow down the pace of the lesson and help to focus student attention.

Pause for reflection also significantly improves student metacognition to develop comprehension.

Creating a pause before or after a comment and raising or lowering one's voice are techniques that can also help to distinguish between essential and peripheral information. After the pause, ask the student to reflect on what they heard. Remember, the whole purpose of the note taking, pausing, and reinforcement is to promote long-term retention.

SUMMARY OF NOTE TAKING

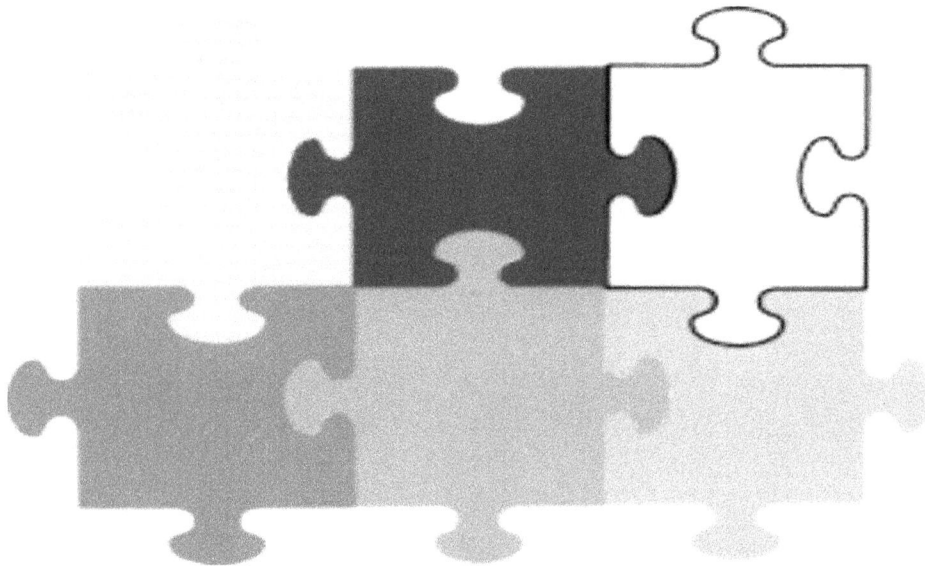

Figure 4.9 Putting it all together.

Top left: Standards used to develop the lesson

Top middle: Student Learning Target (SLT) (in student friendly terms)

Top right: Demonstration of Student Learning (DSL)

Bottom left: Instructional Activities used to meet the Student Learning Target

Bottom middle: Formative Assessments planned

Bottom right: Summative Assessments planned.

Reflection: Do I Have All the Pieces of the Puzzle Planned?

Table 4.5 Sense and Meaning Matrix

Does NOT make sense	*Makes sense*
Has meaning	*Has NO meaning*

Table 4.6 Fix-It Box

It does not make sense because:	*It does not have meaning because:*
I need the following to help me make sense:	*I need the following to help me make meaning:*

Table 4.7 Fixed Box

The information makes sense because	The information has meaning because

Table 4.8 Notes Summary Review

Notes	Make Sense	Have Meaning	Comments Reflection

REFERENCES

Angelo, T. A., and Cross, K. P. (1993). *Classroom Assessment Techniques: A Handbook for College Teachers* (2nd ed.). San Francisco: Jossey-Bass.

Bligh, D. (2000). *What's the Use of Lectures?* San Francisco: Jossey-Bass.

Bloom, Benjamin S. (1956). *Taxonomy of Educational Objectives*. Boston: Allyn & Bacon.

Bloom, B. S. (1976). *Human Characteristics and School Learning*. New York: McGraw-Hill.

Bonwell, C. C., and Eison, J.A. (1991). *Active Learning: Creating Excitement in the Classroom*. Washington, DC: George Washington University.

Caine, R., and Caine, G. (1997). *Unleashing the Power of Perceptual Change: The Potential of Brain-Based Teaching*. Alexandria, VA: Association of Supervision and Curriculum Development.

Davis, O. L., and Tinsley, D. (1967). Cognitive objectives revealed by classroom questions asked by social studies teachers and their pupils. *Peabody Journal of Education, 44*.

Dewey, J., and Boydston, J. A. (1965). Education from a social viewpoint. *Educational Theory, 15*, 73–104.

Hattie, J. A. (1992). Measuring the effects of schooling. *Australian Journal of Education, 36*(1).

Higbee, Kenneth. (1977). *Your Memory: How It Works and How To Improve It*. Englewood Cliffs, NJ: Prentice Hall.

Hill, J. D., and Flynn, K. M. (2007). *Classroom Instruction That Works with English Language Learners*. Alexandria, VA: Association for Supervision and Curriculum Development.

Hunter, R. (2004). *Madeline Hunter's Mastery Teaching: Increasing Instructional Effectiveness in Elementary and Secondary Schools* (rev. ed.). Thousand Oaks, CA: Corwin Press.

Jackson, Y. (2011). *The Pedagogy of Confidence: Inspiring High Intellectual Performance in Urban Schools*. New York: Teachers College Press, Columbia University.

Marzano, R. T., Marzano, J. S., and Pickering, D. J. (2003). *Classroom Management That Works: Research-Based Strategies for Every Teacher*. Alexandria, VA: Association for Supervision and Curriculum Development.

McREL (2005). Research into Practice Series: Classroom Instruction That Works: A Practitioner's Manual for Classroom Instruction That Works. School Improvement Network, Sandy, Utah.

Pintrich, P. R., Smith, D.A.F., Garcia, T., and McKeachie, W. J. *A Manual for the Use of the Motivated Strategies for Learning Questionnaire* (Report No. 91-B-004). Ann Arbor: Regents of the University of Michigan, School of Education, National Center for Research to Improve Postsecondary Teaching and Learning, 1991

Senge, Peter. (2006). *The Fifth Discipline*. New York: Doubleday.

Thorndike, P. W., and Hyes-Roth, B. (1979). The use of schema in the acquisition and transfer of knowledge. *Cognitive Psychology, 11*.

Tomlinson, C., and McTighe, J. (2006). *Integrating Differentiated Instruction and Understanding by Design: Connecting Content and Kids*. Alexandria, VA: Association for Supervision and Curriculum Development.

Willis, J. (2006). *Research-Based Strategies to Ignite Student Learning: Insights from a Neurologist and Classroom Teacher*. Alexandria, VA: Association for Supervision and Curriculum Development.

Wood, E., Prissley, M., and Winne, P. (1990). Elaborative interrogation effects on children's learning of factual content. *Journal of Educational Psychology, 82*.

About the Author

Dr. Mario C. Barbiere has administrative experience at all district levels, as well as college (associate professor) and State of New Jersey level. He has extensive experience in school turnaround, beginning with serving as network turnaround officer for two inner-city schools in New Jersey that had been low performing. Working with the principal and teachers, both schools doubled their test scores in one year and became higher-achieving schools.

Following that, Dr. Barbiere was executive director for Regional Achievement Center, Region 5, created to work with low-performing schools or schools with an achievement gap. Under the Every Student Succeeds Act (ESSA), the Regional Achievement Centers were identified as Comprehensive Support and Improvement (CSI) teams, and Dr. Barbiere served as the regional executive director for CSI 3, covering seven counties in New Jersey.

Dr. Barbiere's doctoral studies were in brain research and lesson design. The research developed interest in instructional delivery and student self-regulation.

Having the opportunity to work in a variety of schools, Dr. Barbiere is passionate about teaching and student empowerment so students are empowered and self-dependent not teacher or school dependent.